KT-416-180

Please return or renew this item by the last date shown. You may return items to any East Sussex Library. You may renew books by telephone or the internet.

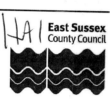
East Sussex
County Council

**0345 60 80 195**  for renewals
**0345 60 80 196**  for enquiries

**Library and Information Services
eastsussex.gov.uk/libraries**

04593920

*of related interest*

**A Pocket Guide to Understanding Alzheimer's
Disease and Other Dementias, Second Edition**
*Dr James Warner and Dr Nori Graham*
ISBN 978 1 78592 458 3
eISBN 978 1 78450 835 7


**Reducing the Symptoms of Alzheimer's Disease and Other Dementias**
**A Guide to Personal Cognitive Rehabilitation Techniques**
*Jackie Pool*
ISBN 978 1 78592 578 8
eISBN 978 1 78450 992 7


**Dear Alzheimer's**
**A Diary of Living with Dementia**
*Keith Oliver*
*Foreword by Professor Linda Clare and Rachael Litherland*
ISBN 978 1 78592 503 0
eISBN 978 1 78450 898 2


**Will I Still Be Me?**
**Finding a Continuing Sense of Self in the Lived Experience of Dementia**
*Christine Bryden*
ISBN 978 1 78592 555 9
eISBN 978 1 78450 950 7


**What The Hell Happened To My Brain?**
**Living Beyond Dementia**
*Kate Swaffer*
ISBN 978 1 84905 608 3
eISBN 978 1 78450 073 3

# Dementia

## Support for Family and Friends

### Second Edition

**Dave Pulsford and Rachel Thompson**

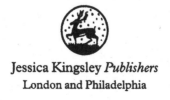

Jessica Kingsley *Publishers*
London and Philadelphia

First published in 2020
by Jessica Kingsley Publishers
73 Collier Street
London N1 9BE, UK
and
400 Market Street, Suite 400
Philadelphia, PA 19106, USA

*www.jkp.com*

**Library of Congress Cataloging in Publication Data**
Names: Pulsford, Dave, author. | Thompson, Rachel, author.
Title: Dementia : support for family and friends / Dave Pulsford and Rachel
Thompson.
Description: Second edition. | London ; Philadelphia : Jessica Kingsley
Publishers, 2020.
Identifiers: LCCN 2019010582 | ISBN 9781785924378
Subjects: LCSH: Dementia--Patients--Care. | Dementia--Patients--Family
relationships.
Classification: LCC RC521 .P85 2020 | DDC 616.8/31--dc23 LC
record available at https://lccn.loc.gov/2019010582

**British Library Cataloguing in Publication Data**
A CIP catalogue record for this book is available from the British Library

ISBN 978 1 78592 437 8
eISBN 978 1 78450 811 1

Printed and bound in Great Britain

# Contents

# Acknowledgements

We would like to say a special thank you to the following people, both people with dementia and family carers who kindly shared their personal experiences and agreed for their quotes to be used in this book. This has provided a valuable insight into the experience of dementia, which we hope will help others.

Previous contributors: Maureen Evans, Kate Harwood, Barbara Pointon and Peter Watson.

New contributors: Jayne Goodrick, Wendy Mitchell, Chris Norris, Keith Oliver, Chris Roberts and George Rook.

# Introduction

## About this Book

This book is for anyone who wants to know more about dementia and how to support those who are affected by this condition. Our readers may be close family members of someone living with dementia, their husband, wife, child or grandchild. Perhaps you have taken on or are anticipating the role of 'main carer' for the person. Alternatively you may be a close friend and want to support the person and their family. You may even have concerns about yourself. How are you feeling at this moment? We are guessing you may be feeling worried and uncertain. This is understandable. However, with guidance and support, some of the fears associated with dementia can be reduced.

Whatever your relationship to the person, we hope you will find this book informative and practical in offering advice and suggestions as to how to help someone with dementia live as positively and fulfilled as possible, whilst also supporting yourselves and each other. Above all, we hope that we can assist you in taking on a positive attitude towards living with dementia. Although being a family member or friend of a person with dementia can be difficult, and sometimes heart-breaking, it can also be positive and fulfilling. With your help and that of others, including paid carers and professionals, the person with dementia can have a good quality of life and experience a sense of well-being right up to the end of their life. This means that you can take some comfort and satisfaction in knowing that you have done your best for the person and those close to them, as well as enjoying the time you have with them as much as possible.

Dementia is a progressive and life-limiting condition for which there is as yet no cure. However, there is much that can be done to help people with dementia. We assume in this book that our readers are committed to making life for a person with dementia the best it can be, but need knowledge, skills and positive attitudes in order to do so. Important aspects of knowledge include information about the type of dementia the person has, how dementia will affect the person and others, and what sources of outside or professional support are available. Understanding is needed of how people with dementia experience the condition, what their feelings are likely to be and, importantly, how they experience the world through the cognitive difficulties that are the main feature of dementia. We believe that the ability to empathise is a particularly important factor in successfully supporting a person with dementia. Important skills include being able to communicate effectively with someone with dementia, helping the person keep active and independent, and responding effectively if the person's behaviour creates challenges.

Also, as dementia progresses, there will be many decision-making points, where either the person themselves or those close to them must decide on future courses of action. We believe the information and ideas in this book will assist our readers with decision-making, and wherever possible, encourage them to include the person with dementia in coming to decisions. We also address the legal underpinnings of supporting people with dementia in the UK. The content derives from our experience as practitioners, teachers and researchers in the field of dementia care. We also bring in the voices of people with dementia, family members and friends, which illustrate their lived experience.

Dementia is a progressive condition that may take years to reach its conclusion. We have adopted the approach of partially structuring this book to reflect its progressive nature. In Part 1, we offer an overview of dementia and what it means to be a family member or friend of a person with dementia. We begin in Chapter 1 with dementia itself and general information about its nature. Chapter 2 covers the fundamental principles of caring for and supporting a person with dementia. Chapter 3 discusses how dementia may begin and the process of assessment that can lead to a diagnosis of dementia. We also consider some of the specific types of dementia. Chapter 4 summarises sources of professional and informal support for people with dementia and their families, and also discusses financial benefits that may be available.

Part 2 concentrates on issues that may arise as dementia progresses. In Chapter 5 we focus on the early signs of dementia, when the person retains many of their abilities and the main role of family members and friends is to help the person retain independence whilst planning for the future. In Chapter 6 we consider how dementia may progress, and how the person's increasing difficulties mean that maintaining independence may be problematic and the person may require more active care and support. In Chapter 7 we reinforce this by considering how people may remain sociable and active as dementia progresses. Chapter 8 is devoted to the challenges of dementia, and in Chapter 9 we discuss the issues surrounding long-term residential care: whether or not to seek a residential care place for the person, how to choose a care home, and how to support the person living in a care home. Chapter 10 addresses advanced dementia, when the person's difficulties are such that they require more or less complete care from others, whether family members and friends or professionals. Finally, as dementia is a life-limiting condition, we contemplate end of life in Chapter 11. Specific issues are discussed within the book at the point in the journey through dementia that they are most likely to arise, but it must always be remembered that people with dementia are all individuals, and the condition may progress and affect people in different ways.

Our focus is on general principles of care and support that can be applied to people with dementia worldwide, but when considering such matters as care and support services and legal and financial matters, we focus on the situation in the UK. We provide web addresses for relevant organisations in the UK in the Resources section at the end of the book.

'Understanding more about dementia and knowing what to expect has helped me know how to respond and cope better.' (Family member)

## PART 1

# Living with Dementia

# CHAPTER 1

# Becoming Familiar with Dementia

## WHAT IS DEMENTIA?

Dementia is a condition that results from diseases of the brain. In medical terms, dementia is a *syndrome* – that is to say, a set of difficulties that the person experiences that can result from a number of underlying causes. Over a hundred different types of dementia have been identified – fortunately, the majority of them are extremely uncommon. In most cases dementia does not affect a person until later in life – the majority of people with dementia are 65 or older – but some diseases that lead to dementia can affect younger people. The most common types include dementia caused by Alzheimer's disease, vascular dementia, dementia with Lewy bodies (DLB) and fronto-temporal dementia (FTD). We will describe these and other forms of dementia in Chapter 3.

People can live with dementia for a long time, so supporting their quality of life is essential. Getting a diagnosis as early as possible enables individuals and their families and friends to understand their condition, reduce and manage risks, plan for the future and make the most of living for as long as possible. This will be discussed in more detail in Chapter 3. It is important to recognise that dementia is a progressive and life-limiting condition which will, in most cases, lead to increasing cognitive difficulties and dependence on others. How long the person will live depends on the type of dementia, their age and general health, but many will live with the condition for several years. Eventually, whilst a person with dementia may die as a result of the condition, some may develop other illnesses that can lead to death, particularly if the person is older. This makes dementia particularly difficult for family members and friends – they have the pain of seeing someone they know and love change and deteriorate, and also need to come to terms early on with the probability of eventually losing that person. It also means that it is important to think about and plan for the future, and although this can be hard to face, it is an issue that needs addressing (see Chapter 5).

People with dementia are not all the same, and individuals will have their own particular difficulties. There are a number of reasons for this:

- As stated above, there are many types of dementia, and these may have different features from each other, especially early on.

- As dementia is a progressive condition, some features are more obvious in the earlier years whilst others appear more as time goes on.

- Factors in the person's make-up will influence how dementia is manifested, including their personality, life history and physical and mental health.

- The way the person is interacted with and cared for by family members, friends and professionals can have a big effect on how dementia progresses.

We will consider these factors in more detail in subsequent chapters.

## FEATURES OF DEMENTIA

Overall, the main difficulties that arise as a result of dementia include memory difficulties, changes in cognitive abilities, problems with communication, changes in emotions or manner and physical changes. All of these can lead to changes in the person's behaviour, and their responses to their difficulties will be significantly influenced by their awareness.

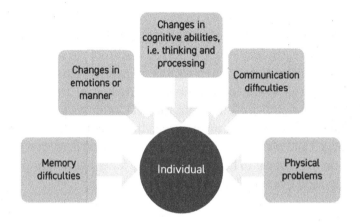

## Memory difficulties

Often, but not always, these are the first signs of dementia. The person may begin to forget things that they would normally have no trouble remembering. Initially, these are likely to be memories of recent events, or newly learnt information. The person might forget someone's name, or what they did the previous day. They might say something as part of a conversation, and then soon after say it again, forgetting that they had already done so. If they are told something new, they might not remember it, or they might find it hard to keep up with what is going on around them. The important thing is that this is a *change* from the way the person is usually – all of us have memory lapses from time to time, and memory difficulties are only a sign of dementia if the person's memory seems significantly worse than it used to be and other changes are also apparent.

'I was renowned for having a brilliant memory, I didn't forget. Then it started to let me down badly and faces and voices became unfamiliar.' (Person with dementia)

'It was particularly my husband's memory; he was continually asking me what the time was, what date it was, what we were going to be doing. He previously would have been more in control.' (Family member)

As dementia progresses, memory difficulties are likely to worsen. In early dementia, the person is still able to remember familiar information, such as the names of close family members, or where to find things in the home. The person can also remember events from the past, often as far back as childhood. As time goes on, however, these memories become damaged and may eventually be lost. In advanced dementia the person may appear to have little memory for either new or past events, and live their life entirely in the present.

## Changes in emotions or manner

The first sign of some types of dementia may not be memory loss, but apparent changes in the way someone feels about things and their manner or outlook on life. Some people may seem to be more inclined to touchiness or anger than is usual for them, whilst others may seem quieter and more subdued, or more anxious about events. These signs may not be recognised for what they are, and family members and friends of the person may think that they are depressed or under stress. This can often happen with younger people who have dementia (those aged 65 or below), as changes in manner and behaviour are common first signs of some of the conditions that affect these age groups.

Such changes may become more noticeable as dementia progresses, and may be reflected in the person behaving in distressed ways, such as becoming very agitated or perhaps resistive and even aggressive in certain situations. Some individuals can become very emotional and cry or become much more upset than they used to. Others may become apathetic and disinclined to do things, and may be depressed. Individuals are very variable, however, and some people may show few changes in personality or in their usual mood.

'I became more irritable, especially when there was a lot of noise when I was concentrating. My family noticed this, of course. My neighbour remarked that I had lost some social awareness and propriety, making inappropriate comments.' (Person with dementia)

'Granddad would describe grandma as being quite stubborn and awkward and those were things that I just couldn't picture in her.' (Family member)

## Changes in cognitive abilities

*Cognitive* means the person's thinking or intellectual abilities. Dementia affects the person's cognitive abilities in many ways. Family and friends will notice the person finding it harder to do many things that they used to be able to do. The person's general thinking abilities may decline – if, for example, they used to be good at crosswords or maths problems or pub quizzes, they may find them increasingly difficult. The person's attention span might reduce, and they may progressively find it harder to concentrate on things for more than a brief period of time, or to attend to things outside their immediate field of view. Their judgement may be affected and they may find it harder to make decisions. This may lead to them sometimes wanting to do things that might risk harm to themselves or others. One example of this is where a person believes that they are still able to drive a car without any problems when, in fact, they are at risk of getting lost or having an accident.

Another thing that can decline is the person's ability to carry out tasks that involve a sequence of actions, such as getting dressed or making a cup of tea – psychologists call this 'impairment of executive function'. The person may put their clothes on in the wrong order or be unable to button their shirt. Ultimately this can lead to people losing the ability to look after themselves, needing help with eating and drinking, keeping themselves clean and going to the toilet.

'The first thing I noticed was losing the ability to be quite as organised as I was... I was noticing more and more that I needed a list.' (Person with dementia)

'I was teaching my wife how to play dominoes and she had no clue that you had to match the numbers together. I thought that was really strange. One day my wife found she couldn't make sandwiches. She was just stood there with two pieces of ham and four pieces of bread, not knowing what to do.' (Family member)

It is not unusual for individuals to try and cover up any difficulties they are experiencing, particularly in the early period, and it may take a while for families and friends to recognise changes. The person may make excuses in order to avoid taking on tasks or finding themselves in situations where they feel exposed. Alternatively, they may relinquish activities to family members in order to make life easier.

'I have given up managing money, since I have lost the ability to make good choices. My wife now looks after our bank accounts and most of my pensions, and our payments, and I am very happy with that as it is one less stress to deal with.' (Person with dementia)

'I could see that my husband's confidence was ebbing away. He even came to me one day as he couldn't work out how to wire a 3-pin plug properly; this was a man who used to construct electronic equipment from scratch.' (Family member)

Yet another effect of memory and cognitive difficulties is *disorientation*. This is where the person has problems knowing where they are or finding their way about, understanding the concept of time, or being able to recognise other people. Disorientation tends to become more pronounced as the condition progresses, and eventually the person appears to lack understanding of the world around them.

'I think one of the first things I noticed was when we were on holiday staying in a hotel and my wife couldn't find her way back to the room. I did think it was a bit odd but I didn't really think much about it at the time... I just thought she was being stupid.' (Family member)

'I became disorientated in a shop once early on, hadn't a clue where I was.' (Person with dementia)

With some types of dementia, difficulties can be encountered with such matters as visual or spatial perception – the ability to follow things visually or to understand how things relate to each other in the physical world. The physical environment may seem distorted to some people, making them anxious when walking about, or the person may not be able to distinguish items from their background. For example, a person may not be able to recognise food on a plate, if the colour of the plate is similar to the food.

'My main problem is trying to distinguish what are memories and what are memories of dreams. I get very mixed up between fact and fiction, dreams and reality.' (Person with dementia)

## Communication difficulties

The impairment of memory and cognition that comes with dementia often shows itself by the person having problems communicating with and understanding others. This can be a particular problem for people with certain types of dementia that affect the parts of the brain that control language and speech (see Chapter 3). Usually in early dementia the person can understand what others are saying, but may find it hard to express themselves in a clear way. Initially, the person's difficulty might be in finding the right name for something (this may include very familiar words such as 'dog' or 'coat'). This can become more pronounced if someone is tired or distracted, and can fluctuate.

In more advanced or specific dementias that affect speech (semantic dementias), the person may find it hard to put together sentences that are understandable to others, even though the person knows what they want to say (the term that psychologists use for this is 'expressive dysphasia'). This is obviously very frustrating for the person and hard for those family members and friends with whom the person is trying to communicate.

> 'I think and speak more slowly. It takes little distraction to stop me finding words and thoughts. Noise destroys me. I cannot take part in normal group conversations as I cannot keep up with speakers and respond in time to keep conversations going.' (Person with dementia)

> 'One time mum couldn't get her words out and she got upset and she lashed out at me. It was as though she wanted to tear her hair out, she was in such a state and I had to hold her hands and say, "Don't do that to me mum, I'm only trying to help you. I hate what's happening to you." And she ended up getting upset and I got upset too.' (Family member)

Sometimes, what the person says can reflect difficulties in their thinking or perception. The person may develop a firm belief that something is true when it really isn't. This may mean that they are misinterpreting things, or it could be what psychologists call 'delusional thinking'. This can cause distress for the person and their family and friends, such as when the person firmly believes that others are stealing things from them, or that their mother, for example, is alive and coming to visit, when, in fact, she died many years ago. It is important to understand that in many cases this kind of thinking is a result of people trying to make sense of the world around them in the context of their fading memory and thinking abilities, and creating a reality that helps them to cope. It can also stem from the person mixing up memories of the past with the present.

A common difficulty experienced in communication is that people with dementia become repetitive and may ask the same questions again and again, or utter the same phrases many times over. Much of the time this occurs as a result of memory loss and the person will have simply forgotten they have said something a few minutes before.

'The first sign was that grandma would repeat herself, ask the same question again or say the same thing over and over again.' (Family member)

Other people may hear voices in their heads or see things that aren't actually there ('auditory or visual hallucinations'), and talk as if they were real. In some types of dementia this can be a significant feature. It is also not uncommon for older people to experience problems with their eyesight, which, if not corrected, can lead to visual misperceptions. It is important to establish the cause and recognise that these experiences are part of the condition. We will discuss how to respond to such communication issues in Chapter 6.

As the condition becomes advanced, the person may seem to lose the ability to understand what others are saying to them – we say 'seem to' because by this point the person may have lost the ability to talk meaningfully to other people and so we can't really tell if they can understand us or not. It may well be that the person still understands something of what we are saying to them – it is likely they will pick up on the feelings behind the words that we are uttering and be comforted or distressed according to what those feelings are. Again, we will say more about how to communicate effectively with people with advanced dementia in Chapter 10.

## Physical problems

As we have discussed above, dementia is a progressive condition, and as it becomes advanced, the person may experience noticeable physical decline. There are a number of physical changes that may develop as the condition progresses, including problems with eating, drinking, using the toilet and walking. In addition to this, some types of dementia have physical symptoms such as poor balance throughout their course as well as the psychological symptoms that we have been describing (see Chapter 3).

> 'My balance is terrible and I have many injuries and scars from falling, which affects your confidence in getting about.' (Person with dementia)

## OTHER CONSIDERATIONS
### Reduced awareness

'Awareness' refers to the extent that the person with dementia is aware that they have the condition, and understands the effects that dementia is having on them. People vary in how aware they are. In early dementia, some people have considerable awareness of their condition and its implications. This allows them both to take action to compensate for their difficulties and to make plans for the future when their level of awareness will be reduced. With others, awareness declines from the outset and the person may deny that there is anything wrong with them. This can create problems for family members and friends as the person may not accept their help, or may insist on carrying on with activities that they are no longer able to perform safely.

As dementia progresses, awareness tends to decline along with the person's cognitive ability, and the person may lack understanding of why others are not letting them do certain things, such as going out of the house on their own, or they are apparently insisting on doing things to them, such as making them have a wash or go to the toilet.

### Changes in behaviour

It will be apparent that the person's memory, emotional and cognitive difficulties are likely to lead to considerable changes in the ways that the person behaves and acts. We have mentioned that the person will find some abilities declining, leading them to do less than they did before. The person may also start to behave in different ways and do things that may be hard for others to understand, such as hiding away or hoarding things or having a strong need to walk about. Sometimes the person may behave in ways that family and friends find very challenging, such as being extremely irritable or agitated. Such behaviour may often seem random and inexplicable, but as we will see in Chapter 8, it may well have meaning for the person.

'I have problems with keeping myself under control sometimes; I tend to say what I think straight away. A tap on the arm from my wife stops me now, but it might not in the future.' (Person with dementia)

'I thought my husband was doing it deliberately; he used to take my oven gloves and throw them on top of the kitchen cabinet where I couldn't get them. Instead he was hiding them safely because he knew they were important and shouldn't get lost. I thought he was being difficult.' (Family member)

## THE EXTENT OF DEMENTIA

Whilst dementia can affect people at any age, it is by far most common in older people, and the longer you live, the greater chance you have of developing it. Few families have been unaffected by dementia, and it may be helpful for readers to know that they are far from alone in having to come to terms with it. A report published by the Alzheimer's Society in 2014 estimated there were 850,000 people living with dementia, with this number set to rise to 1 million by 2025. At the same time, dementia is not just an issue for industrialised societies – despite generally lower life expectancy, the large majority of people with dementia live in developing countries. In 2015 Alzheimer's Disease International estimated that 46.8 million people worldwide are living with dementia and that numbers are expected to double every 20 years. This is obviously significant in financial terms, with the worldwide costs of dementia, according to the *World Alzheimer Report 2015*, being US$818 billion, and projected to be US$1 trillion by 2018. It is said that if dementia care were a country, it would be the world's 18th largest economy.

Dementia is not, however, an inevitable consequence of growing older – only 7.1 per cent of all over-65s in the UK have dementia. The following table sets out prevalence rates for dementia in the UK for each age group:

| Age group, years | Male (%) | Female (%) |
|------------------|----------|------------|
| 30–59 | 0.16 | 0.09 |
| 60–64 | 0.9 | 0.9 |
| 65–69 | 1.5 | 1.8 |
| 70–74 | 3.1 | 3.0 |
| 75–79 | 5.3 | 6.6 |
| 80–84 | 10.3 | 11.7 |
| 85–89 | 15.1 | 20.2 |
| 90–94 | 22.6 | 33.0 |
| 95+ | 28.8 | 41.1 |

Less than 10 per cent of those below the age of 80 will have dementia, and less than a fifth in their 80s will be affected. It will be no comfort to those with dementia in their family to know that they are in a minority, but there is no inevitability that even if we live to 100 that we will develop dementia. As we will see later, there is growing evidence that our risk of developing dementia can, to some extent, be reduced by some simple lifestyle changes.

## WHAT CAUSES DEMENTIA?

All forms of dementia are ultimately caused by damage to, or loss of, brain cells (neurons). In the various types of dementia, different areas of the brain are initially affected, leading to the range of signs and symptoms characteristic of each condition. The actual mechanisms by which brain cells are damaged are complex and poorly understood, but overall, three broad 'risk factors' for dementia can be identified:

- *Increasing age:* As we have seen above, the most common types of dementia are all 'late-onset', affecting people after the age of 65, so the longer you live, the more likely it is that you will be affected by dementia. At the same time, there are many rare conditions that lead to 'young-onset' dementia (before the age of 65), and the risk of developing these reduces as you get older.

- *Genetics:* Why does one person develop a medical condition whilst another of the same age and with an apparently similar lifestyle does not? Doctors assume that this is due to differences in their genetic make-up. Genetic factors certainly play a significant role in whether or not a person will develop dementia. However, genes work in complex ways, and except for a few extremely rare conditions, it is not the case that if your parent(s) had dementia you are inevitably going to develop it as well (or vice versa). Scientists have identified a number of genes that in conjunction with each other may increase or decrease an individual's risk of dementia. However, the complexity of our genetic make-up means that it is not possible to predict who will, or won't, develop dementia, unless you have a rare form of dementia in which a faulty gene is inherited.

- *Lifestyle:* There is growing evidence that factors in our lifestyle may, to an extent, raise or lower our risk of dementia, and as with other medical conditions, an interaction of genetic and lifestyle factors determines our risk profile. We consider these factors in the next section.

## CAN DEMENTIA BE TREATED, CURED OR PREVENTED?

Our first thought on hearing that someone we are close to has an illness is, can it be treated or cured? The blunt answer to this question as far as dementia is concerned is that with our current state of understanding there is no cure for any type of dementia, although researchers offer hope that this situation may change. There are some drugs that offer short-term relief of symptoms for Alzheimer's disease dementia, and new drugs that may further delay the progression of dementia are under development. In addition, research is beginning to identify ways in which lifestyle can be adapted to slow down the progression of the disease. We will discuss these in Chapter 3.

### Reducing the risk of dementia

There is growing evidence that aspects of our lifestyle may influence whether or not we will develop dementia and how it progresses. As we will see in Chapter 3, there is clear evidence that cardio-vascular factors are present in the most common types of dementia that affect people in later life, and a lifestyle that may protect against cardio-vascular diseases such as hypertension (high blood pressure), diabetes, heart attack and stroke may also protect against dementia. Simple healthy behaviours such as avoiding smoking, drinking alcohol within safe limits, maintaining recommended body weight and eating a 'Mediterranean diet' – minimising red meat and saturated fat and including plenty of fruit and vegetables and oily fish – are as relevant to preventing dementia as they are to warding off other illnesses. Maintaining regular exercise into old age is also important, with strong research evidence that moderate exercise done on a regular basis may reduce the risk of dementia.

Another factor that appears to influence dementia is educational engagement, and in particular, maintaining intelligence-based activity into old age. If we continue as we grow older to carry out mind-stimulating activities such as reading, crosswords and puzzles, learning new things and playing musical instruments, we may delay the onset of dementia or at least keep our brains active and stimulated enough to help slow deterioration. However, be wary of 'brain training' books or computer packages that advertise their ability to ward off dementia. None have a firm evidence base, and keeping up a generally social and mentally stimulating lifestyle into old age is likely to have a greater protective effect than carrying out specific brain training exercises once in a while.

In short, there are things we can do to reduce our own risk of developing dementia. A recent study has concluded that up to one-third of cases of dementia could be prevented if people adopted the lifestyle changes set out above. There is also some evidence that treating cardio-vascular factors such as high blood pressure and high cholesterol, helping the person remain physically active and promoting cognitive stimulation may help slow the progression of dementia in those who have the condition. Whilst there is much still to be learnt about dementia, and we are many years away from eradicating it, we are not completely helpless in protecting ourselves and those people with dementia who are our family members and friends from the worst effects of the condition.

## DEMENTIA IN SELDOM-HEARD GROUPS

Dementia can potentially affect everyone, but it is important to consider the particular issues and needs of those groups that do not make up the majority of people with dementia.

### Different seldom-heard groups
#### Young-onset dementia

The majority of cases of dementia are classed as 'late-onset', defined as dementia that manifests itself when the person is over the age of 65. Dementia can, however, affect people at any age, and a proportion of people will have young-onset dementia. This is sometimes also called 'early-onset' or 'working-age' dementia, and it is when the signs of dementia appear before the person has reached the age of 65. In the UK, around 40,000 people have young-onset dementia (it should be noted that this figure is likely to be an under-estimate, due to misdiagnosis of symptoms).

> 'I was still working and dementia was the last thing I thought of – it had never entered my vocabulary.' (Person with dementia)

Sometimes the disease process is the same as for late-onset dementia, but often different diseases with their own particular features lead to young-onset dementia – we will overview some of the more common conditions in Chapter 3. Young-onset dementia carries its own particular challenges for the person, family and friends and professionals. The person has more to give up – they are more likely to have a job and may have child-rearing and financial responsibilities that will have to be taken on by other family members whilst also caring for the person with dementia. A younger person with dementia may be more physically fit and active, which means that it can be harder to meet their needs for activity, and can lead to more acute problems if the person's behaviour causes difficulties to others. Also, the rarity of young-onset dementia can lead to issues with providing professional support services or residential care. As there will be comparatively few people with young-onset dementia in a particular geographical area, it can be hard to provide specific services, and younger people may be forced into services designed for older adults due to lack of more appropriate alternatives. This can be compounded by the fact that different forms of young-onset dementia have very different features to each other, leading to experts suggesting that services for younger people should be specific to the type of dementia – which is even harder to provide for small numbers of people. However, there is growing awareness of the specific needs of younger people with dementia, with recent developments in research and specific organisations and services emerging that are trying to meet needs and influence policy.

'Younger people with dementia have specific needs – we are often here for the long haul as we might be physically fitter, we may be working or have to leave work early which has financial considerations and some people still have children to look after. But we also have a lot to contribute.' (Person with dementia)

## Black, Asian and minority ethnic (BAME) groups and dementia

There are at present an estimated 25,000 people from BAME groups in the UK who have dementia, and it is predicted that the prevalence of dementia in these groups will increase at a much faster rate than in the white British population. This is because the overall age profile amongst BAME groups is currently younger than the population as a whole. The challenges of dementia amongst BAME groups are considerable. There is evidence that some groups, such as those from South Asian (Indian, Pakistani and Bangladeshi) and Black Caribbean backgrounds, are at higher risk of developing dementia due to higher rates of hypertension and diabetes. There is, however, a lack of understanding of dementia amongst some groups – there is no word for dementia in some South Asian languages – and the signs and symptoms of dementia may be attributed to normal ageing or to mental illness. This can lead to families not seeking help in a timely fashion. Other factors may discourage families from BAME groups from accessing services. Amongst some groups (for example, South Asian and Chinese groups) there may be cultural pressures on adult children to look after parents with dementia, whilst BAME groups in general may feel (sometimes with good reason) that health and social care services that cater mainly for the white British population may not be able to meet their cultural or religious needs. This is not helped by the lack of culturally sensitive diagnostic tools and difficulties with accessing interpreters.

These perspectives may be mirrored by the attitudes of service providers. There is often an assumption that BAME families do not need professional help, as 'they prefer to look after their own'. This may be the case amongst traditional South Asian or Chinese families, but there is evidence that younger generations amongst these groups are taking on more 'Westernised' attitudes. Also, many older people from Black Caribbean backgrounds live alone. Professionals may underestimate the stress and difficulty of caring for a person with dementia from a BAME background, believing that extended families will come together to reduce the burden, but research has shown clearly that being a carer is stressful regardless of ethnic background or family make-up. Finally, the overt or hidden discrimination that people from BAME groups face on a day-to-day basis can make caring for a person with dementia even more complicated. As with young-onset dementia, there is a growing awareness of the specific needs of BAME groups, and in some areas efforts are being made to offer bespoke services.

**People with learning disabilities and dementia**
There are strong links between learning disabilities such as Down's syndrome and dementia. People with learning disabilities are at a higher risk of developing dementia, and tend to develop it at an earlier age than the population as a whole. In the past this was less of an issue, as people with learning disabilities tended to have relatively low life expectancy. Today, medical advances and improved social care have lengthened life expectancy for people with learning disabilities, leading to growing numbers with dementia. As with other groups, Alzheimer's disease is the most common cause of dementia, and its prevalence increases with age, but people with learning disabilities develop the condition 20 or 30 years before the population as a whole.

It might be thought that dementia is less problematic for a person with learning disabilities as they already have some cognitive difficulties. However, dementia can lead to profound negative changes in the person's cognitive abilities, which may mean the person becoming more disabled than before, and can cause as much distress to the person's family and friends as with anyone else who develops dementia. It can also, as with others, shorten the person's life expectancy. Recognising dementia in a person with learning disabilities can be difficult as they are already having cognitive difficulties, and it may be that changes in mood and behaviour are noticed first. It is recommended that those who have an understanding of learning disabilities carry out specific assessments, and that specialist support is offered.

### Lesbian, gay, bisexual and transgender (LGBT+) people with dementia

Around 6 per cent of the UK population regard themselves as LGBT+ and therefore it is likely that a similar percentage of people with dementia will be LGBT+. Readers who are a family member, partner or friend of a lesbian, gay, bisexual or transgender person who develops dementia will face the same issues as anyone else. However, in some ways the experience of LGBT+ people with dementia can be different to those who are heterosexual or cisgender, particularly when it comes to interacting with professionals who may lack understanding of their needs or even be aware of their situation. LGBT+ people may be more likely to become detached from their families, leading to fewer sources of support if they develop dementia, or increased reliance on partners or friends. They may have hidden their sexuality for years, and they and their partner may not feel able to be open with professionals about the true nature of their relationship, which can lead to the needs and potential contributions of their partner being ignored by professionals. Some who have worked in residential care have had the experience of a resident being visited regularly by a 'close friend' of the same sex without realising that the friend was the resident's partner – or thinking to ask the visitor if that was the case. Also, some professional carers, particularly in residential care, may harbour negative attitudes towards LGBT+ people, which may affect the care the person is given.

Transgender people with dementia may also face other challenges in addition to the above. For example, there is some evidence that transgender people with dementia may revert to their previous gender identity, and older people may face health problems related to the gender they were assigned at birth; for example, a transgender woman may, in later life, experience prostate problems. Dementia may make such issues harder to identify and treat.

There is increasing awareness of the needs of LGBT+ people living with dementia, and some areas are beginning to develop specific services to meet their needs and offer support.

## Families and friends of seldom-heard groups

If you are a family member or friend of a person with dementia who fits into one of these seldom-heard groups, you may recognise some of the extra challenges that this implies. We will discuss specific issues relevant to these groups as this book progresses. However, the goals of dementia care and the principles of supporting a person with dementia are the same regardless of the person's circumstances. Quality of life and well-being are still paramount, and understanding how to assist the person in attaining these goals is key to supporting the person in their journey through dementia. At the same time, having an understanding of the specific issues with dementia amongst these groups can help family members and friends anticipate and manage those issues if they arise. Particularly important is establishing a proper dialogue with professionals, who may sometimes themselves need educating regarding the needs of people with dementia from seldom-heard groups. Sources of information and support available for those from seldom-heard groups who have dementia are listed in the Resources section at the end of the book.

## WOMEN AND DEMENTIA

Whilst the impact on men of developing dementia or becoming a carer to a person with dementia should not be underestimated, dementia is predominantly an issue for women, with research showing that women feel the impact of dementia more than men. As the prevalence of dementia increases with age and women overall live longer than men, the majority of people with dementia in the UK are women – 69% women compared to 31% men. Women are also much more likely to take on the role of main carer for a person with dementia; two-thirds of unpaid carers are women, and women are more likely to take on tasks such as personal care. Women carers report that they feel less supported in the caring role than their male counterparts, perhaps because other family members and friends feel that a woman can manage the role more easily and willingly. At the same time, women may be less inclined to seek support, although they may find it easier to talk about their experience of being a carer (and we suspect they may be more likely to purchase books such as this one). Women of working age are more likely than men to reduce their hours or give up work altogether to become a carer, with both financial and life satisfaction implications. Finally, the large majority of professional carers for people with dementia are women and they are likely to receive less pay than men in equivalent roles.

This state of affairs mirrors the experience of women in society as a whole, and there are no straightforward solutions. Female readers may be slightly comforted by the knowledge that they are not alone, and should use that knowledge to demand more of their male family members and friends. Male readers should not assume that caring is automatically a female role and should recognise female carers' needs for support. Ultimately, political action is needed to reduce the persistent gender gap in the UK and elsewhere.

## A RIGHTS-BASED APPROACH TO DEMENTIA

People with dementia and their carers have the same needs and rights as anyone else but may feel discriminated against at times. People with other disabilities have demanded human rights and equality, and there is now recognition that dementia should be viewed in the same way. A number of organisations have produced statements to support the need for a rights-based approach. The National Dementia Action Alliance (NDAA) is a body that brings together organisations across England to share best practice and take action on dementia. It has published a set of 'Dementia Statements' compiled by people with dementia and their carers that highlight the fundamental rights of people with dementia and those who support them:

- We have the right to be recognised as who we are, to make choices about our lives including taking risks, and to contribute to society. Our diagnosis should not define us, nor should we be ashamed of it.

- We have the right to continue with day-to-day and family life, without discrimination or unfair cost, to be accepted and included in our communities and not live in isolation or loneliness.

- We have the right to an early and accurate diagnosis, and to receive evidence-based, appropriate, compassionate and properly funded care and treatment, from trained people who understand us and how dementia affects us. This must meet our needs, wherever we live.

- We have the right to be respected, and recognised as partners in care, provided with education, support, services and training that enables us to plan and make decisions about the future.

- We have the right to know about and decide if we want to be involved in research that looks at cause, cure and care for dementia, and be supported to take part.[1]

---

1    https://nationaldementiaaction.org.uk/dementia-statements/

These statements show that thinking about dementia has come a long way since the time when people with dementia were regarded as having few rights beyond basic physical safety, and long-term institutionalisation was the predominant means of providing support. The clear message today is that people with dementia are people like ourselves who, with support, can have a good quality of life and contribute to society.

# CHAPTER 2

# Being a Family Member or Friend of a Person with Dementia

- How does it feel knowing that someone close to us has a long-term progressive condition?

- How will our relationship be affected as the condition progresses?

- What should our role be as a family member or friend?

These are difficult questions to consider but they are important in preparing for the inevitable changes to come. As dementia progresses, the person is likely to need increasing support, not just with meeting their daily living needs, but also for maintaining a sense of well-being. And that means they rely on family and friends.

How do we feel about being in this crucial but demanding position? Our initial reaction to dementia may be negative. We may be filled with a sense of foreboding when we think of the changes ahead and the emotional and physical demands they may cause. We may experience a gradual and continuing sense of loss as the person we know starts to change. That sense of loss may even make us want to distance ourselves from the person.

Alternatively, for some, it may be an opportunity to become closer through having a new role of providing support and care, and being able to spend time together in a way that wasn't required before.

> 'I have had to adjust my whole manner of being with my husband; where responses used to be natural and automatic, I now have to halt my immediate response and second-guess the reaction I may or may not receive.' (Family member)

The experience of dementia for families and friends will inevitably be influenced by the quality or nature of our previous relationships. Some people may find themselves in a caring role due to a sense of love and willingness, whilst others may feel ambivalent or even resentful. Whatever the relationship, the ability to understand and adjust to changes and develop coping strategies has an important influence on how we feel and respond. This will also impact on the person we care for. For couples in particular, the ability to share feelings and thoughts and negotiate decisions is crucial in maintaining relationships. This may become more difficult as the condition progresses or if the person has little awareness of their condition. If the previous relationship was negative, this will also present a significant challenge. However, the opportunity to talk about feelings of loss, frustration and ambivalence, and how to cope, can be extremely helpful.

As the person's understanding of the world diminishes, the familiarity of family and friends becomes more and more important. Even in advanced dementia, when the person may not recognise those closest to them, the emotional comfort that only the presence of a loved one can provide will help them experience a measure of well-being. This is not to suggest that family and friends should be morally obliged to take on all the work of caring for a person with dementia. Caring for a friend or family member who has dementia can be very stressful, particularly when behaviour changes, and it is not a role everyone feels they can take on.

Professional carers who have the right understanding and skills can provide much-needed emotional comfort and support. Professional help is important at all phases of the journey through dementia (see Chapter 4), and as we will discuss in Chapter 9, residential care may eventually be the most appropriate option for some people with dementia. Family members or friends can sometimes feel guilty for having failed in some way if they hand over direct care, but even if the person goes to live in a care home, the ongoing contributions of family and friends should not be underestimated.

## FAMILY, FRIENDS AND BECOMING A 'MAIN CARER'

Supporting a person with dementia places considerable responsibility on family and friends, and it is a responsibility that some will feel better able to take on than others. Many people with dementia want to live in the community in familiar surroundings and with familiar people, and many families want that for them as well.

It is common for a particular person, usually a close family member or sometimes a friend, to take on the role of 'main carer'. That person may do most of the work of caring, they become the person that the individual with dementia most relates to, and are often the one liaising with professional services. Sometimes the main carer takes on the role voluntarily and would prefer that they had that role rather than other family members. Sometimes, however, a person can become the main carer by default, because they are the person's only relative, or other family members are unable or unwilling to take on the responsibility and subtly (maybe sometimes unsubtly) push another into the caring role. In such circumstances, it is not surprising to learn that women are more likely to take on the role of main carer to a person with dementia than men. Such family dynamics are perhaps inevitable but clearly place the bulk of the caring responsibility onto one person, who may feel unsupported or abandoned if other family members or friends then step back and leave them to it. It should be the responsibility of family members and friends that the 'main carer' is not abandoned in this way.

## THE GOALS OF SUPPORTING A PERSON WITH DEMENTIA: QUALITY OF LIFE AND WELL-BEING FOR ALL

We mentioned in the Introduction to this book that by family members and friends supporting a person with dementia, the person may achieve the best quality of life and sense of well-being as possible. What do these concepts really mean, and how can family members and friends help a person with dementia reach these goals? How can they also maintain their own well-being and quality of life?

'Quality of life' and 'well-being' are rather vague concepts but ones that we can apply to ourselves. We could all make a list of those things that we feel enhance our quality of life and make us feel good – folk music, red wine, country walks and meals out with our families and friends feature highly on our own lists! In early dementia, when the person still retains many of their abilities, there is no reason why their lives cannot broadly continue as before and they can derive well-being from their accustomed activities and pastimes. As the person's range of abilities starts to narrow, however, some preferred activities might, on the face of it, become difficult or perhaps seem impossible. However, a person with dementia will still derive well-being from the same broad aspects of experience as we all do.

The following figure highlights some aspects that can be particularly important for people with dementia and their carers in maintaining well-being and quality of life (adapted from the IDEAL project).[1]

---

1    www.idealproject.org.uk

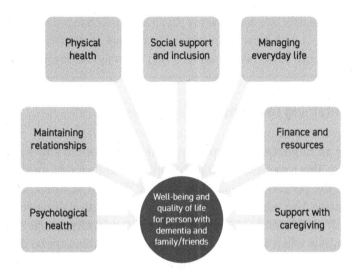

## Psychological health

We will all undoubtedly agree that this is important to our own sense of well-being. Anxiety or depression, which often accompany dementia, will have a negative impact on well-being, and supporting someone's psychological health may require treatment and support from health care professionals (see Chapter 4). However, there are things we can do that can make a significant difference to psychological health. The psychologist Tom Kitwood suggests that attention to the person's needs for comfort, inclusion, identity, attachment, occupation and love is important for people with dementia. Receiving affection, dignity and respect can significantly contribute to well-being. It can take as little as an aggressive driver sounding their horn at us unnecessarily to put a cloud on our day, and arguments and ill-feeling within the family will make us feel bad. People who have dementia are no different. As dementia progresses, the ways that family members and friends interact with the person are put into sharper perspective, with little things that others say and do having a strong influence on the person's sense of well-being or ill-being (see Chapter 6).

> 'I have difficulty with how my physicality has changed towards him – I withdraw involuntarily and have to overcome my reticence when he just wants a hug.' (Family member)

## Maintaining relationships

Supporting someone to maintain positive relationships will have an important influence on their quality of life and well-being. This may be through maintaining your own relationship with the person, although this may be difficult at times, and ensuring the person is able to maintain relationships with family and friends. Although sadly some family or friends withdraw when someone develops dementia, this may be due to their own misunderstanding and worry about how to be with that person. We provide some useful suggestions about helping people to maintain relationships in Chapters 5, 6 and 7. Many people with dementia derive great pleasure from meeting and being with other people with dementia. Chapter 4 includes information about support groups that can assist them to do so.

> 'I've lost some friends; some people don't know how to talk about it; some don't believe it. But for every friend I've lost, I've gained three through all the peer support groups and activities I'm involved in as a result of my dementia.' (Person with dementia)

## Physical health

Anyone who has experienced a serious illness will be aware of the negative impact it can have on well-being and quality of life. The same is the case for people with dementia. Ensuring physical health problems and medication are monitored is essential, and the person may need help and encouragement with attending regular health checks. As indicated in Chapter 1, managing our lifestyle, diet and exercise can be vital ways of reducing risk of further deterioration. Keeping as active as possible can also be important in maintaining quality of life and well-being. We all know that exercise can make us feel both physically and emotionally better. Many people with dementia will have been active throughout their lives and will want to keep active as their dementia progresses. This may simply take the form of being on their feet and walking about, or it may, at some level, reflect the desire to continue leisure or work activities that the person once enjoyed. Although this may be more of a challenge as dementia progresses, supporting someone to stay active and/or adapting exercise so they can stay as active as possible will be important for their health, well-being and quality of life.

'Since giving up work four years ago, keeping physically active, walking my dog and gardening are really important to me.' (Person with dementia)

## Social support and inclusion

Many activities also imply socialising with others. One of the strongest contributions that family members and friends can make to enhance the well-being of people with dementia is to help them feel socially included, either by assisting them to keep up with pastimes that they previously enjoyed or by finding new things that the person can do despite their difficulties. Above all, people want to feel included and involved, irrespective of how dementia is affecting them, and the more we can do to enable this, the better it will be for the person. Indeed, people with dementia are increasingly talking about the importance of 'living as well as possible with dementia', but may need support to do so.

'I believe "doing" keeps my dementia at bay. Being exposed to different conversations in different environments keeps my brain challenged.' (Person with dementia)

## Managing everyday life

Many people with physical disabilities have a strong need to maintain independence and to do things for themselves rather than have others do things for them. Those with cognitive difficulties as a result of dementia, are no different. This may, in early dementia, be reflected in a desire to continue to live independently, and giving up that independence can be difficult. As dementia progresses, maintaining independence is linked to keeping active – the more the person can do for themselves, whether it is helping around the house, pursuing hobbies themselves or simply getting themselves washed and dressed, the more they are maintaining a level of activity. Also, such activity, requiring an element of thinking for themselves, helps provide cognitive stimulation, which may help slow the progression of dementia. It may be that people will need supervision or indeed get things 'wrong', but the opportunity to stay involved is vital.

> 'My grandma will walk over to the supermarket every day to get the things she needs...that's her pleasure, that's the only thing she does. If we take away going to the supermarket from her, she'd have no quality of life.' (Family member)

### Making choices

Being independent implies choosing how to live our lives. In early dementia the person is likely to retain considerable capacity for making choices about their life. There may be times, however, when reduced awareness or insight may result in the person making choices that are not in their best interests, such as refusing help or wanting to continue activities that put them at risk. In these situations, the role of family and friends in supporting the right choice is extremely important and can require great skill and diplomacy. As well as helping the person make choices in the present, family members and friends can assist them to make choices about their future, through drawing up *advance statements* or *advance decisions* (sometimes known as 'living wills') regarding what the person would want when they cannot make big decisions for themselves (discussed in Chapter 5).

As dementia progresses, major decision-making may be very difficult for the person, but offering choices should not be ruled out completely. It will enhance dignity and respect for the person if we ask them what their choice would be where possible rather than deciding for them, even if it is as simple a matter as 'would you like tea or coffee?' or showing them a couple of options for food or clothes to wear.

'I want to manage my dementia proactively rather than reactively, so it's important to me that I make choices whilst I can, and that people know what I want in the future.' (Person with dementia)

### Familiarity and continuity

People with dementia will often feel more secure and content in an environment that is familiar and with a routine that maintains continuity and minimises major changes. This is partly because more long-standing memories are retained better than recent memories, so the person may recognise things and people that remind them of long-term aspects of their life and derive comfort from that recognition. Also, whilst people with dementia can adapt to new environments and learn new things, too much change and unfamiliarity may be hard for them to take in and come to terms with. Family members and friends can assist a person with dementia experience familiarity simply by their presence, as people the person knows and loves. They can also contribute to promoting a familiar environment for the person even if they have to move to residential care, by passing on their knowledge of the person and their life to care staff, or by making the person's living area more like home by bringing in some of their furniture, possessions or photographs.

## Finance and resources

Having some financial security and resources clearly has an important impact on all of the above. Many studies suggest that a lack of finance can be an important factor on people's ability to continue providing care. Whilst we have no magic solutions for this, we would urge readers to ensure they seek advice and support from local authorities and/or voluntary sector agencies about possible available benefits (see Chapter 4). Equally important is the need to ensure financial procedures are put in place to help someone manage and protect their money before they lose the capacity to do so. This is explained in more detail in Chapter 5.

## Support with caregiving

It will be evident, however, that as dementia progresses the person will need more and more assistance from others with managing their lives as their range of abilities changes. As time goes on, the balance between promoting independence and doing things that the person cannot do for themselves will shift. At all times, the person will need a level of help to compensate for their cognitive difficulties. Ultimately this may include providing assistance with basic needs such as eating, drinking and keeping clean. To what extent this help will come from family and friends or from professional carers will depend on a range of factors, but whether or not the person is receiving full-time professional care, family members and friends will have a role to play in helping to ensure that the person's needs are met. As we have suggested, though, people often need support with caregiving, and it is important to seek help rather than 'soldiering on' alone. In order to support a person's quality of life and well-being, we also need to look after our own quality of life and well-being. This may include emotional support, practical advice, developing new skills, practical support with providing care, an increased understanding and/or developing coping strategies. We discuss below important ways of looking after oneself.

## THE QUALITIES NEEDED TO SUPPORT A PERSON WITH DEMENTIA

What personal qualities do family members and friends need to support someone with dementia and assist them to achieve well-being and a good quality of life? In our view, three broad qualities are needed in helping to provide a compassionate approach. These are: the ability to empathise with the person, a positive attitude and supporting and caring skills.

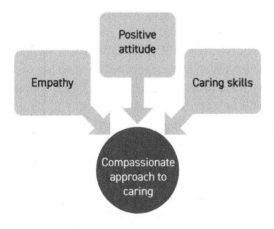

### Empathy with the person with dementia

Family members and friends should attempt to empathise with the person, by trying to appreciate how the person is feeling and also, importantly, how the person understands the world around them through the screen that their cognitive difficulties places between them and their world. In other words, this involves trying to 'step into their shoes'. Psychologists call this *cognitive empathy* – understanding how another person is thinking and their perspective on the world. If we can achieve this, we can help the person in more than one way. First, we can assist the person to manage their life by finding ways of compensating for their cognitive difficulties, just as we help people who have physical difficulties. Second, by recognising that the person's actions or words reflect their cognitive difficulties, we can avoid blaming the person when they do or say things that we may find frustrating or upsetting – we can with honesty say to ourselves that 'they can't help it' and seek to find ways of reducing such misunderstandings or minimising their effects on others.

## A positive attitude

In the past, society had an almost totally negative view of dementia. This stereotype can be traced back to Shakespeare's description of decrepit old age in *As You Like It* as 'second childishness and mere oblivion, sans teeth, sans eyes, sans taste, sans everything'. When faced with the reality of dementia, however, we need to attempt to transcend such thoughts. How we do so will be very individual. For many of us it will be a simple question of continuing concern for someone who has been important to us and who we love. Others may approach the issue from the perspective of how they would want to be cared for if they themselves developed dementia. However we do it, supporting a person with dementia begins with the assumptions that the person is still a person worthy of our respect and love and that we can make a positive difference to the person's quality of life and sense of well-being.

## Caring skills

Supporting or caring for a person with dementia is a skilled business. We need to know how to interact and communicate with the person, how to help them manage their difficulties whilst maintaining their independence, and how to respond when their behaviour creates challenges for us. We also need to adapt our approach as the person's condition progresses. There is no reason to suppose that we will already possess these skills – why should we if we have not known a person with dementia before?

## UNDERSTANDING THE NATURE OF DEMENTIA

The personal qualities set out above rely on family members and friends having an understanding of the nature of dementia. This understanding must be at several levels. First, we need to understand the condition itself. As we will discuss in the next chapter, it is important that a diagnosis is made and that family members and friends know what that diagnosis is, what it implies for the person and how the condition is likely to progress. We need to know if any medical treatments are available and what effects they might have. We also need to know what might be the consequences for the person's ongoing physical health as well as their cognitive state.

Second, we need to understand the specific effects that dementia is having on the person and the actual cognitive difficulties that the person is experiencing. The cognitive difficulties that people with dementia develop may affect their ability to manage their lives in two broad ways. They may *misunderstand* the world around them, including other people. If a family member or friend says something to the person, they may misinterpret it, or just not understand it at all. As discussed in Chapter 1, the person may not recognise who is talking to them, even if it is a close family member or friend. Similarly, they may misinterpret aspects of their environment, such as reading the weather wrong or failing to recognise where they are. For some people there can be visual-spatial difficulties – problems with judging distances or interpreting visual signs or cues. It is also possible for someone to develop false perceptions or hallucinations – seeing or hearing things that are not really there and responding to them as if they were real – or false beliefs or delusions – believing something to be true and responding accordingly.

The other way that people with dementia may experience cognitive difficulties is through reduced ability to *respond* to the world around them. The person may understand what has been said to them but may not be able to find the right words to answer. They may know where they are but be unsure of how to get to where they want to go. They may see and recognise a cup, kettle and packet of tea bags on the kitchen shelf but can't work out how to make a cup of tea. If asked to decide on something, they may understand the issues but lack the ability to put those issues together to make a decision. The figure below summarises the main cognitive difficulties that dementia can cause, divided into these two broad categories.

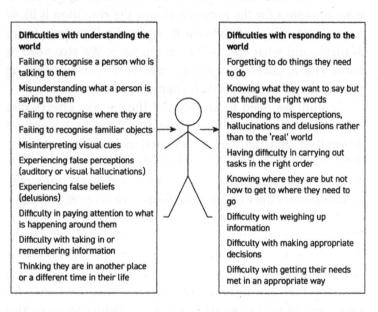

**Difficulties with understanding the world**

Failing to recognise a person who is talking to them

Misunderstanding what a person is saying to them

Failing to recognise where they are

Failing to recognise familiar objects

Misinterpreting visual cues

Experiencing false perceptions (auditory or visual hallucinations)

Experiencing false beliefs (delusions)

Difficulty in paying attention to what is happening around them

Difficulty with taking in or remembering information

Thinking they are in another place or a different time in their life

**Difficulties with responding to the world**

Forgetting to do things they need to do

Knowing what they want to say but not finding the right words

Responding to misperceptions, hallucinations and delusions rather than to the 'real' world

Having difficulty in carrying out tasks in the right order

Knowing where they are but not how to get to where they need to go

Difficulty with weighing up information

Difficulty with making appropriate decisions

Difficulty with getting their needs met in an appropriate way

Put together, these difficulties lead to the person displaying what we commonly term 'confusion'. Confusion is a blanket term for behaviour, speech or manner that comes from the person either misunderstanding the world around them or not being able to respond appropriately to the world around them, or both. It is important for family members and friends to look beyond the rather stark term 'confusion' and to try to work out what the specific difficulties are that the person has with relating to the world.

Understanding the basis of the person's cognitive difficulties is the key to empathising with the person. If we can, as it were, get inside the head of the person with dementia and appreciate how they perceive the world around them, if we can recognise when the person can respond appropriately to events in the world and when they can't, we can come up with ways of helping the person compensate for their difficulties.

'I try to understand and not comment when he forgets, or becomes lost. It's easier if we can ignore the difficulty, instead of highlighting a mistake.' (Family member)

## INDEPENDENCE VERSUS ASSISTANCE

One of the most difficult aspects of supporting someone with dementia is balancing offering assistance whilst maintaining the person's independence. When helping a person with dementia compensate for their cognitive difficulties, family members and friends sometimes have a difficult balancing act to perform. On the one hand, we want to ensure that the person gets their needs met quickly and appropriately. On the other hand, we should be aiming for the person to be as independent as possible. As we have seen, independence carries lots of benefits for a person with dementia: it helps keep the person active, it enhances well-being and it may even slow the progression of dementia. This means that family and friends should be trying to assist the person with dementia to do things for themselves, and only do things for the person if it is clear they are unable to do those things unaided. A simple analogy can be made with physical disability. Suppose a person has weakness in their legs and finds it hard to stand up out of a chair. If we see the person struggling to rise, we are tempted to go over and help them up. Our motivation for doing so is often twofold: first, we want to make things easier and less effort for the person, and second, we want to reduce the risk of the person falling and coming to harm. The same motives lie behind our wanting to do things for a person with dementia. Often it can seem easier to do something for the person, such as tidying their house, making them a cup of tea or, in the later phases, getting them dressed rather than watch them slowly struggle to do so themselves. Also, we sometimes see genuine risks in the person being independent, of them accidentally coming to harm, or even being exploited or abused by others. Balancing the risks of independence with the benefits is one of the hardest tasks for those supporting a person with dementia, and deciding when to intervene and take away an aspect of independence can be very difficult, especially if the person does not see the risks.

> 'I responded by taking over everything that he appeared to struggle with. I disabled him far earlier than the dementia did, but out of love and wanting to make things better.' (Family member)

> 'My husband's very restless and wants to go out and walk around all the time. I used to do this with him but I've accepted I can't go with him all the time now so have to "take the risk" and hope that he'll be safe. But as he gets more confused about the time of day I expect this will get more difficult.' (Family member)

## THE IMPACT OF DEMENTIA ON CHILDREN

Dementia affects the whole family, and it is important not to forget the impact it can have on children. Children will often experience dementia through contact with a relative (or the relative of a friend) who has dementia. This is usually a grandparent (or great-grandparent, as more people are living to their 80s or 90s), but it is also possible that one of their parents may develop young-onset dementia.

Dementia can affect children in a number of ways. They may become aware of changes in the person and their relationship with the person altering. Perhaps a grandparent who gave them lots of attention and treats gradually becomes more inward-looking and less inclined to make a fuss of them. Sometimes children may notice the person speaking or behaving in ways they find hard to understand. Also, dementia can increase strains within a family, as when a hard-pressed parent has to care for their own parent with dementia as well as look after their own children. Children are very sensitive to their parents' emotions, but may struggle to understand why their grandparent (or parent) is acting the way they do and why their mum or dad is getting so stressed and upset.

The best approach is to be open with children about the fact that the person has dementia. How this is done will depend on the age of the child and the nature of their relationship with the person. Generally there will not be a need for too much detail, but some books and online resources are available that aim to explain dementia to children and young people if they want to know more, for example an animation produced by Dementia UK (see the Resources section at the end of the book) that shows how dementia might affect someone and how children can still maintain an important role in the person's life. Important points are that the person has an illness of the brain that affects the way they think and talk and that sadly will get worse. Also be open about how it affects you and how it can make you stressed and upset. Let the child ask questions and reassure them that the person with dementia still loves them and can't help it if they seem less loving than they used to.

Such an approach, done sensitively, should reassure the child and get them on your side when caring for the person. People with dementia often like and respond well to children, and a relationship with a child who has an awareness of the person's condition and is used to their manner and behaviour can be fulfilling for both.

'Our children's reaction has been mixed. One has shown an absolute, natural, instinctive understanding and ability; another has buried his head and keeps away. He is not able to deal with what he perceives may happen.' (Family member)

'My youngest grandson has only been told quite recently that I have dementia, but I think he had twigged. When he was told he just accepted it.' (Person with dementia)

## THE ROLE OF PEER AND PROFESSIONAL SUPPORT

A key aspect of supporting a person with dementia is to have support oneself for undertaking that role. This support should come both from within the family and one's circle of friends, and also from professional services. We stated earlier that in many cases a particular person becomes 'main carer' for the person with dementia, either willingly or by being more or less thrust into that role. Some of our readers will be in this position, whilst others will be more concerned with remaining in touch with the person with dementia and supporting the main carer. Whatever your role, a positive attitude towards the person with dementia needs to be accompanied by a positive desire to support one another. Accepting help and support from others is essential, both practically and emotionally, whatever your relationship with the person with dementia.

'What you need is someone to talk to face-to-face, a hug when you are down, or somebody to say "You are doing fine, you are okay". Encouragement keeps you going.' (Family member)

'It isn't just the spouse or the family that need support; friends also need support. My friend and I have given each other an enormous amount of support and she has come along to some of the education groups since, which have helped her.' (Family member)

Professional care and support should be available for people with dementia at all its phases, but access to professional support and the quality of professional input are ongoing issues for people with dementia and their families and friends. There is debate about how much the government should pay for dementia care and how much the cost should be borne by the person with dementia and their family. At its best, professional input can make an important contribution to enhancing the well-being of people with dementia and easing the challenges for families and friends. Whilst specific service provision varies from place to place, we will discuss in Chapter 4 the main types of professional support available.

## FAMILY MEMBERS AND FRIENDS: LOOKING AFTER ONESELF AND EACH OTHER

Being a family member or friend of someone with dementia will place emotional and sometimes practical demands on an individual and will require considerable personal skills and qualities. Caring is a demanding role for which few people have been given any preparation or training, and which will carry continual responsibility for a considerable period of time. A key difference to other caring roles is the impact that dementia has on the person's cognitive abilities and manner and subsequent relationship change. Looking after oneself and each other is crucial for maintaining well-being, for both carers and people with dementia alike.

> 'I never thought of myself as a carer; it wasn't a profession I ever wanted or was trained for. I worked with children with special needs, but it's different when it's in your personal life.' (Family member)

There is little 'rocket science' behind the principles of looking after oneself. Carers of people with dementia cope with the demands placed on them in the same way that they have become accustomed to coping with other demands throughout their lives. Everyone has their own way of managing situations and emotional demands, and it is often a matter of recognising that you are in need of emotional support and reaching for familiar coping strategies. Key principles of personal and mutual support include the following.

### Talking with others

Having an outlet for your feelings, thoughts and anxieties is always useful. Being able to talk about your situation with trusted family members or friends will help keep that situation in perspective. Alternatively, support groups or internet forums may provide opportunities to talk with others in similar positions.

'I have been lucky as I've had a really good friend; we have just talked for hours and hours.' (Family member)

## Being available to others

It is important that family members and friends do not avoid contact with the person with dementia or with their main carer. Sharing the caring role makes that role easier, and being able to interact with a range of family members and friends will help enhance the quality of life of the person with dementia.

'It all started with a good friend over the road who walked a dog. He said, "Do you think your husband will come round the village with me when I walk the dog?" So I said, let's try it. And this is how it began. Then other dog walkers and habitual strollers met them on their rounds, and people in the village formed a rota to accompany my husband on his walk every day – enabling him to enjoy the fresh air and me to have a bit of respite from the constant vigilance.' (Family member)

## Recognising stressors

Carers need a good measure of self-awareness, to recognise when their feelings of anxiety or stress are becoming too much. It is important to acknowledge that there will be times when you feel under pressure. It is also important to recognise that we are not superheroes – we cannot do everything or get everything right; we can only do what we can.

'I had to ask the GP what to do as I was a bit at my wits' end.' (Family member)

## Taking time out

It can be tiring and sometimes frustrating being with a person with dementia (or indeed anyone) for an extended period of time. As dementia progresses, people may have increasing needs and anxieties and they may follow you around, sometimes asking the same questions many times. Using empathy, we can recognise that this reflects the person's uncertainty about themselves due to their memory loss and lack of ability to orientate themselves to what is happening around them. But we may still become frustrated with the person, and this frustration could boil over. Better to take 'time out', have a cup of tea and let our feelings subside.

## Taking breaks and holidays

If you are a full-time carer of someone with dementia, try to give yourself regular breaks and holidays. Friends and other family members could assist by volunteering to stay with the person whilst you go out for the evening or take a holiday. Support services such as day centres or respite care may be employed. It is a good idea if on a respite break to avoid the temptation felt by many carers of people with dementia to continually check that the person is okay, by phoning the respite facility or even visiting the person there – a break should be a break.

'Having time for me was really helpful; having time to do something different; being able to do what I wanted to do.' (Family member)

## Keeping up with hobbies and interests

Breaks and respite periods may, of course, be used for carers' own hobbies and interests, and it is important that carers make time during the day for things they like to do.

'Dad played bowls a lot and he enjoyed it and it was a bit of time for himself. We didn't want dad to give up his bowling, so

> during the bowling season we would, between us, have mum with us so she had someone with her.' (Family member)

## Using support services

As we have said, support services can sometimes appear to be thin on the ground during the early years of dementia, but it is important that carers know how to access them.

> 'I think I would benefit from having time to deal with my emotions; I tend to hide from it all and then collapse in a heap. I get very angry with my husband sometimes and I know I shouldn't, but it makes me feel bad. If I could work these things through with someone, I think it would help us both.' (Family member)

## HOW THIS BOOK CAN HELP

Our aim in this book is to assist family members and friends in acquiring the understanding and caring skills they need in order to support a person with dementia and themselves. We provide basic information about the main types of dementia and their ongoing effects. We try to help readers appreciate the difficulties of dementia and learn to empathise with the person's feelings and understanding of their world. We try to enhance readers' skills at interacting with people with dementia in a range of situations, and outline sources of professional support and how to access such support.

What we can't do is give our readers a positive attitude towards people with dementia. That has to come from within.

# CHAPTER 3

# Someone Close to Me May Have Dementia

## Assessment, Diagnosis and Types of Dementia

### IDENTIFYING DEMENTIA

- Do you know for sure that someone close to you has dementia?

- Has the person undergone a formal assessment process and been given a diagnosis?

If so, it is likely that you will already be familiar with much of the information contained within the early sections of this chapter. You may have gone through a period of uncertainty when the person's cognitive abilities gradually appear to decline, have undergone the stressful process of assessment and cognitive testing, and have eventually received the news, expected or otherwise, that it is dementia. The difficult journey will have begun, but you will know what is happening and will have some idea of what to expect.

At the same time, whilst awareness of dementia is increasing, due to public health campaigns and enhanced specialist assessment and diagnosis, some people with dementia never receive a formal diagnosis. If you suspect that a person you are close to may have dementia but are unsure what to do next, this chapter may help you understand what is happening to the person and encourage you to seek a proper assessment and diagnosis. As we will see as we go through the chapter, there are significant advantages of doing so.

## THE FIRST SIGNS OF DEMENTIA

Many conditions that have far-reaching consequences for the person and those close to them begin with small and apparently trivial signs, and dementia is no exception. Dementia characteristically starts with the person making little mistakes or acting in ways that are a bit unusual for them, but not especially alarming.

We all sometimes act in ways that mimic the earliest signs of dementia. Consider whether you have ever...

- Forgotten an appointment?

- Made a cup of tea and then forgotten you have made it?

- Found it hard to find the right word for a familiar object when in conversation?

- Not been able to identify the day of the week?

- Forgotten the name of a person you know?

- Lost your way going to somewhere you've been to before?

- Forgotten to pay a regular bill?

- Put something down and not been able to find it again?

- Felt particularly moody or angry and not known why?

- Had problems with concentrating or taking in new information?

We suspect that many of you will have ruefully admitted that some of the above have happened to you at some time. This does not, of course, necessarily mean that you have dementia. You may, however, recognise some of this list as being the first warning signs that all was not well with the person you are now concerned about. The fact that dementia in its earliest phase appears to be little more than day-to-day absent-mindedness can make it very hard for family and friends to realise that something is amiss.

'I was finding it difficult to remember staff names at work, who said what in which meetings, and what had to be done in my calendar.' (Person with dementia)

'It's difficult to say when it started for my mother – at first we thought she was depressed from retiring from work.' (Family member)

Eventually, however, the person's manner and behaviour becomes sufficiently unusual and problematic for family and friends to become concerned. The key to recognising possible dementia may be there is a noticeable *change* in the person. Perhaps someone whose memory is normally spot on starts to become forgetful or a characteristically cheerful person becomes moody or distracted. The change may alternatively be one of degree – a person may have always been somewhat absent-minded or touchy, but becomes noticeably more so.

'I became more irritable, especially when there was a lot of noise when I was concentrating. My family noticed this of course. My neighbour remarked that I had lost some social awareness and propriety, making inappropriate comments.' (Person with dementia)

'My husband had always been in charge of finances, but I went into his office one day and found that he had not being organising his paperwork; things had been opened and not dealt with. I realised he was not taking things in. It was a bit of a shock.' (Family member)

Stereotypes of old age can hinder recognition of dementia. Some images of older people may include becoming slower on the uptake, forgetful and set in their ways. Nothing could be further from the truth about the majority of older people, but if an older person acts in these ways, we may well say 'it's their age' rather than consider the possibility of dementia. For younger people, dementia is not often considered and changes may be attributed to stress, low mood or possible physical causes.

> 'The GP suggested it was depression at first and then migraine, but I knew it wasn't. They didn't think it was dementia because I was young and my symptoms weren't typical.' (Person with dementia)

Another factor that may prevent dementia being identified is what we may harshly call 'denial'. None of us wants to contemplate the possibility of a close relative or friend developing dementia, with all the implications that the condition brings. If a person we love starts to act in the ways listed above, we may make excuses for them, or play down the significance of the way the person's manner is changing. Sometimes this reluctance to face the possibility of dementia can persist long after the signs of the condition are obvious, and the person may either receive a diagnosis when symptoms are more advanced or in some cases never receive a formal diagnosis of dementia. It is important to remember that if there is sufficient concern, this is always worth investigating.

## HOW PEOPLE WITH DEMENTIA REACT TO THE ONSET OF THE CONDITION

People react to the onset of dementia in a range of ways. Some will interpret their experiences of absent-mindedness or moodiness as temporary lapses caused by everyday stresses, or by 'old age creeping on'. Some may look to physical or other psychological causes as the reason. Others will be increasingly aware that all is not well but will downplay the issue through 'denial' or may hide their growing difficulties from family and friends so as not to alarm them. Still others may acknowledge the problem and be willing to seek help.

> 'It was my husband who noticed it and wanted to do something about it. He said, "I'm forgetting things and I think I shouldn't be" – we decided to go to the GP.' (Family member)

A proportion of people with early dementia will have already begun to lose awareness of their condition and will deny anything is wrong with them due to a genuine lack of understanding of what is happening to them. This will create extra issues for concerned family and friends who may notice changes the person doesn't see, and may try to persuade the person to seek help when they don't themselves see the need for it. In such cases diagnosis may be delayed, or the family may find themselves resorting to 'white lies' in order to get the person assessed. If you have concerns but the person or other people are reluctant to get an assessment, it is important to remember that there are significant benefits to getting a diagnosis. Information leaflets about the process and options for treatment and support may be helpful (see the Resources section at the end of the book for further details). Concerns should also be shared with professionals who are responsible for the person such as their general practitioner (GP), as they may have more success in encouraging the person to have an assessment. For older people over the age of 75, an annual general health check provided by GPs now includes a 'screen' or check for signs of dementia, and this may be a useful way to access an initial assessment.

## DIAGNOSING DEMENTIA

Diagnosis is the process whereby a health professional formally confirms that a person has a particular condition and names that condition. Diagnosis allows treatment to be given, if available, and means that a prognosis may be offered – a forecast of how the person's condition may progress and what the future will hold. A diagnosis of a life-changing condition such as dementia is a highly significant event – a watershed in the life of the person and their family and friends – and is as devastating as a diagnosis of cancer. How that diagnosis is obtained will have a significant bearing on how the person and those close to them face the future.

'It was getting harder and harder to do my job, writing, doing reports, etc. I was aware of all the things I couldn't do any more. My family could see the changes and encouraged me to see the GP, so I did.' (Person with dementia)

There is now a systematic process that should be followed to investigate memory or cognitive problems and diagnose dementia. In the first instance the person should consult their GP. In some cases the GP will feel confident to assess and diagnose the person themselves, but if dementia is suspected, they should also refer the person to a memory assessment service (sometimes called a memory clinic). This is a multi-professional service that has the specialised role of assessing, diagnosing and treating such problems. The process of investigating for possible dementia is a systematic one:

- A full medical history of the person is taken, including any previous physical or mental health problems.

- A physical examination is carried out, to rule out any treatable causes of the person's symptoms.

- An initial test or screen of the person's cognitive abilities is carried out.

- The person may be referred for a 'brain scan', otherwise known as an MRI, CT or SPECT scan.

- More in-depth cognitive tests (known as *neuro-psychological tests*) may be carried out to help determine specific types of dementia.

The centrepiece of assessment is the test of cognitive abilities. This will be administered by the assessor, usually a mental health nurse or a psychologist, but may initially be the GP, who will ask the person questions and give the person brief tasks to perform. A range of tests is available for the purpose of assessing possible dementia. Some are very brief and can include between three and ten simple questions. These test a combination of abilities such as recent memory, orientation, calculation, visual-spatial ability (usually through a clock-drawing test), recognition of familiar objects and the ability to retain information. For less typical dementias, longer neuropsychological tests may be carried out that can detect problems with verbal fluency, organisational skills and perception. In addition to these, information should be gathered from a close relative or friend. This ensures that any changes the person themselves are unable to report are noted. If this is not offered, it is important you request this, and it should be carried out separately to the assessment of the person if you are concerned about causing upset or distress.

Cognitive testing is, of course, a very anxiety-provoking process for both the person and those close to them. Although the initial tests are brief and the questions are simple, it is like taking an examination, the result of which will have far-reaching implications. Testing should be carried out in a sensitive and professional way, with the person given every opportunity to give their best performance – a suggestion that someone has dementia when, in fact, they do not will not be helpful.

'Mum was angry – she said, are they testing to see if I'm stupid?' (Family member)

The brief cognitive tests carried out are often not appropriate for people with a different language or cultural background and do not pick up signs of some types of dementia, particularly those with a younger-onset dementia. In these cases, alternative approaches may be required.

> 'I kept passing the test so they told me it wasn't dementia. I spent two years going backwards and forwards to the GP trying to get them to take on what I was saying but I only had success when I went to a different GP and they sent me to the memory clinic.' (Person with dementia)

## Possible outcomes of cognitive assessment

In broad terms, there are four possible outcomes of a cognitive assessment, as indicated in the figure below.

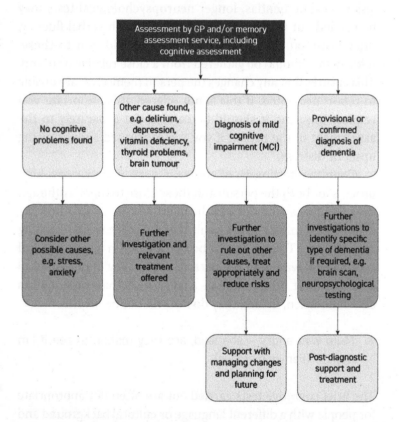

### No cognitive problems found

It is quite possible that the person's cognitive abilities are found to be 'normal' and the person has no indication of dementia. The person's difficulties may be more felt than real, and the assessment will reassure them there is no significant problem. However, it may be useful to consider possible causes for concern such as stress or anxiety, and continue to monitor these in case of future changes or ongoing issues.

### Other cause found

Investigations may reveal another condition is causing the person's symptoms. It may be the person is experiencing *delirium*, a state that can be caused by a number of illnesses in which the person appears to be 'confused' (sometimes called *acute confusional state*). A wide range of conditions can cause episodes of delirium in older people, in particular infections, but also dehydration or constipation. Delirium can often be distinguished from dementia by its sudden onset and fluctuations in behaviour. Treating the underlying condition should relieve the symptoms. Delirium is a significant issue for older people and particularly those with dementia, and a separate section about this is included below.

Another condition that can mimic dementia is *severe depression*. Again, the person may appear to be forgetful and confused, but history taking and sensitive assessment by a professional may reveal that the person is actually very depressed. Treatment of the underlying depression with antidepressant medication and psychological therapies should, in time, lead to the person's cognitive abilities being restored. Some other conditions may also appear like dementia, including some vitamin deficiencies (particularly B12 and D), thyroid problems and brain tumours. These should be investigated and treated to reverse cognitive changes where possible.

### Diagnosis of mild cognitive impairment (MCI)

Assessment of the person's cognitive abilities may reveal some deficits, but not enough for a doctor to say for sure that the person has dementia. In such cases, the person may be told that they have *mild cognitive impairment*. This means exactly what it says: there is evidence of some impairment of the person's cognitive abilities, but these do not normally interfere with daily life. MCI can be caused by a range of factors, including normal ageing, but in some cases it may predict the person will go on to develop dementia. It is not possible with current knowledge to identify with any certainty who will actually do so, although studies suggest only 5–10 per cent of those with MCI will develop dementia. A person diagnosed with MCI may be recommended to prepare for the possibility of developing dementia by setting up a lasting power of attorney (LPA) or drawing up an advance statement or decision (see Chapter 5). Some of the strategies discussed in Chapter 5 to help people manage early dementia may also be helpful to those with MCI.

### Provisional or confirmed diagnosis of dementia

The final possible outcome of cognitive assessment is that a diagnosis of dementia is made. Often a brain scan or in-depth neuropsychological tests are needed to diagnose the specific type of dementia, which may be important in making decisions about treatment options. For those with this outcome, the process of adjusting to and managing dementia has now formally begun for the person and for their family and friends.

## AFTER THE DIAGNOSIS

Research has highlighted what people and their families and friends need at the point of diagnosis. An initial need is for information, about dementia as a concept, about the specific disease that the person has and about what the family and friends require to help the person. Second is the need for access to practical, emotional and social support, for the person and for those close to them, in order to maintain well-being and quality of life. Third is treatment including medication (if relevant), and psychological treatments such as cognitive stimulation therapy or cognitive rehabilitation should be offered that may in some cases slow the progression of the condition and alleviate symptoms (see Chapter 5). Finally, there is the need to plan for the future, as the time will inevitably come when the person will not be able to care for themselves, and will need help and care from others.

Unfortunately, it is not always the case that these needs are met effectively by memory assessment services. These have a role in prescribing and monitoring medication for those for whom they are recommended (see Chapter 5), but for some people with dementia these drugs are not effective, and the person is discharged from the memory assessment service back to the care of their GP. Many people with dementia and their families report being more or less abandoned by professionals once the diagnosis has been made, with little advice or support other than a general 'contact your GP if you have any problems'. People with early dementia and their families and friends are often left to fend for themselves, a state of affairs that is increasingly being regarded as unacceptable in political and professional circles.

> 'Whilst my experience of assessment and diagnosis was very good, I wish I had been given coping strategies at the time. People should be given a care plan at the time of diagnosis to help prepare them for what's to come.' (Person with dementia)

> 'I was given a leaflet but had really nobody to talk to. We were just sort of shown out into the street.' (Family member)

As we will see in Chapter 4, some initiatives are being developed to provide more help for families following diagnosis, and knowing how to access such help is important. But in the rest of this chapter and in subsequent chapters, we will attempt to provide some of the basic information and advice that is needed once the diagnosis of dementia has been confirmed.

## WHY IS DIAGNOSIS IMPORTANT?

Before we move on, it is worth considering this question. If some people with dementia never receive a diagnosis and apparently get through their lives, why is diagnosis so important?

The importance of diagnosis for the person and their family is threefold. First, diagnosis creates certainty – the person's experiences and actions can be explained, understood better and information can be forthcoming. Second, plans can be made for the future – we will talk more about this in Chapter 5. Finally, diagnosis provides access to professional services and to treatment, if available – again, we will discuss currently available treatments below. Professional opinion is virtually unanimous that early assessment and diagnosis of dementia is highly desirable, hence the focus on expanding memory assessment services.

'I think when we were told the diagnosis I felt relief because we'd got a name for what my husband had. I think it was later it became more real. I initially thought, now it's got a name, like measles or mumps, I thought, okay, we can deal with it.' (Family member)

'Without a diagnosis we would have both spiralled into a maelstrom of arguing, of fighting, of lack of understanding, and our marriage may well have died. We would both have been lost to dementia, without even knowing why.' (Family member)

## SHOULD THE PERSON WITH DEMENTIA BE TOLD THE DIAGNOSIS?

This can be a controversial and sensitive question. In the past, it was felt that a person with dementia should not be told about their condition, either because they could not take it in or understand its implications, or because they might find the news overwhelming. The result was often a conspiracy of silence in which family and friends avoided the issue when with the person. Some readers may remember that years ago this was often also the case with people who had cancer – it was common for doctors to give the diagnosis of terminal cancer to the person's relatives rather than the person themselves, and a similar conspiracy of silence would prevail until the severity of their condition became obvious to the person.

'I don't think we ever said the word "Alzheimer's" to mum. I think we said, "Your memory's not good", or something like that. I think I said lots of words about what was happening to her, but not that word.' (Family member)

Today the situation with disclosing a diagnosis of cancer to the person is very different and except in rare circumstances the person will always receive the diagnosis themselves. There is now consensus that the same should, as a rule, be the case for people with dementia. With diagnosis tending to be made earlier, many people retain awareness and can both take in the news and use it in a positive way, by finding ways of compensating for their difficulties and by making plans for the future. To be told that they have dementia is, of course, distressing for the person, and family and friends sometimes want to keep the diagnosis from the person to save their feelings, but research indicates that on the whole people with dementia (like people with other life-threatening illnesses) want to know the truth and can cope with the implications of diagnosis.

'I actually think that the period following diagnosis, black though it was, is a positive... I don't want to go there again, so it spurs me on to do things that are keeping me busy and interested.' (Person with dementia)

'There was a part of me that was pleased to hear a diagnosis. It isn't the end of your life, it's a line in the sand, and then you can think how you're going to live well with whatever you've got.' (Person with dementia)

What if the person appears to lack awareness of what is happening to them? Would it be helpful to try to tell them the diagnosis in those circumstances? This is not a straightforward question. Sometimes people with dementia have more awareness than is apparent and can absorb information despite not appearing to do so. At the same time, if a person has a profound lack of awareness of aspects of their present situation, it may not be helpful to remind them of their reality if it is likely to cause distress. We will return to the issue of responding to different realities that people with dementia can experience later in this book (see Chapter 6).

> 'The diagnosis was very clearly explained to us, but when we were with the doctor I looked round and saw that my husband had gone to sleep; he couldn't cope with any long detailed explanations by that time.' (Family member)

## THE MAIN TYPES OF DEMENTIA

A principal need of people with dementia and their families and friends following diagnosis is information about their condition. In the case of dementia, this means both information about the broad syndrome of dementia (discussed in Chapter 1) and information about the specific type of dementia that the person has, provided that a particular type has been identified. As stated earlier, there are over a hundred types of dementia; as the majority are extremely rare, we won't try to list every one in this book. In this section and the next we will, however, say something about the most common types of dementia.

### Alzheimer's disease

This is the most common cause of dementia and accounts for approximately two-thirds of older people with dementia and a third of those with younger-onset dementia. Dementia caused by Alzheimer's disease has the features that are most frequently associated with dementia. It usually begins with memory problems, the person particularly having difficulty remembering newly learnt information. Memory deficits gradually worsen and other signs start to appear, such as problems with language, orientation, attention and carrying out daily tasks ('executive function'). Changes in mood and behaviour will often occur as a result. The development of difficulties usually happens slowly, over a period of months or years, the person becoming more and more dependent on others.

Alzheimer's disease dementia is a neurodegenerative disorder, meaning that it is caused by the degeneration and death of cells in the brain (neurons), particularly in the cortex, the grey matter that makes up the surface of the brain. This causes the brain of an affected person to *atrophy* – it shrinks, losing weight and volume as cells gradually die. The biochemical processes that lead to the degeneration of brain cells are highly complex and not fully understood. However, two things happen to affected brain cells that together are diagnostic features of this dementia. First, large numbers of *plaques* develop around diseased cells. These are deposits of a protein called 'beta-amyloid' and can be seen under a powerful microscope. Second, *neurofibrillary tangles* are found within the same cells. These are deposits of another substance called 'tau protein', which, under the microscope, appear like tightly tangled threads. Research is still underway to help us completely understand the role of both beta-amyloid and tau proteins in causing brain cell damage in dementia. It is now recognised that the process of neurodegeneration can begin many years before the person starts to show the signs of dementia.

As mentioned in Chapter 1, Alzheimer's disease is the most common cause of dementia in people with Down's syndrome. Typically the age of onset of the condition is earlier than in the population as a whole. The high rate of Alzheimer's disease in people with Down's syndrome is thought to be caused by the presence of extra genes on chromosome 21.

**Treatment and progression of Alzheimer's disease dementia**
As with other types of dementia, there is currently no treatment for Alzheimer's disease that will lead to a cure or stop the continual process of brain cell damage. There are, however, some drugs that may help improve the condition for a time.

There are two types of drugs available for those with Alzheimer's type dementia that can be prescribed following diagnosis by a doctor or memory assessment service. The first type is group of drugs called *acetylcholinesterase (AChE) inhibitors*. These drugs can compensate for the loss of a brain chemical called 'acetylcholine', which plays a role in memory and other cognitive functions. Three drugs are available within this group: donepezil (marketed in the UK as Aricept), rivastigmine (Exelon) and galantamine (Reminyl). These all work in slightly different ways but the benefits can include improvements in thinking, memory, communication or day-to-day activities. Common side effects can include nausea, sleep problems, diarrhoea, muscle cramps or tiredness, but these are often mild and don't last long, and they don't affect everyone. One drug may suit a person better than another due to the way they work or are administered, but some people who take the drugs find that they do not gain much benefit from them. Whilst the AChE inhibitor drugs may be limited in what they offer, many people with dementia and their families appreciate the benefits that they can bring.

Another type is called 'memantine' (Ebixa). This works in a different way to the AChE inhibitor drugs and is recommended for relief of symptoms in people with more advanced dementia or those with moderate dementia when AChE inhibitors are not suitable. Side effects can include headaches, dizziness, drowsiness or constipation, but these are usually short-lived. Again, its benefits are modest, but evidence suggests that it may help make some people feel less agitated and reduce psychotic symptoms (seeing or hearing things) if present.

There are also some psychological therapies that may help people in early dementia delay the progression of the condition, or help them manage its effects. They are not universally available, but an overview is provided in Chapter 5.

Research is being carried out worldwide to try to find better treatments for dementia, but less money is put into dementia research than into other life-limiting conditions such as cancer. Current opinion is that whilst there is unlikely to be a 'cure' for Alzheimer's disease in the near future, treatments that delay or prevent onset are within reach. What is clear is that we are learning more about Alzheimer's and other dementias, and there is hope that further research will lead to new solutions.

The long-term prognosis of Alzheimer's disease, as with other illnesses that lead to dementia, is for increasing difficulties leading eventually to death. How long a person will live with the condition will be very variable, and because many will not show symptoms until very late in life, many will die from other age-related illnesses before dementia becomes advanced. It is quite possible, however, for a person to live for a number of years with the condition.

## Vascular dementia

As the name suggests, vascular dementia is caused by cerebral-vascular disease, that is, disease of the blood vessels, affecting circulation of blood around the brain. Vascular dementia is itself a syndrome, and there are several specific diseases that are included within the term. In all cases, however, vascular dementia is caused by disease or damage to the blood vessels that supply the brain cells, leading to loss of blood supply and consequent damage and death of brain tissue. The three most common forms of vascular dementia are:

- *Multi-infarct dementia:* In this condition, the person experiences a series of 'mini-strokes' or transient ischaemic attacks (TIAs) in which blood supply to the brain is interrupted. Each time the person experiences a TIA, another small area of brain tissue is damaged, causing loss of cognitive function in that area. Eventually, if TIAs happen frequently enough, the grey matter of the brain becomes sufficiently damaged for the signs and symptoms of dementia to become apparent.

- *Single-infarct dementia:* In some cases, a person who has had just one large stroke may afterwards display all the signs and symptoms of dementia, if the stroke occurred in a particular area of the brain.

- *Small vessel disease-related dementia:* Also called 'sub-cortical vascular dementia' or 'Binswanger's disease', this condition results from damage to the blood vessels deep inside the brain. The person may not notice changes, but memory and thinking can be affected over time.

## Vascular and Alzheimer's disease dementia compared

The onset and progression of vascular dementia may vary from that of Alzheimer's disease. Sometimes its onset is relatively sudden, reflecting the fact that the person has had a stroke or a TIA. Sometimes the condition progresses in a 'step-wise' pattern, in which the person may experience an abrupt onset of symptoms followed by a relatively long period of stability. The person then experiences another small stroke that leads to another increase in symptoms, and that pattern continues over a period of months or years until the difficulties become profound. The nature of the person's difficulties may be very individual; unlike Alzheimer's disease, in which there is often a general increase in difficulties in all areas of the person's cognitive life, with vascular dementia some abilities may be profoundly affected early on whilst others are preserved, reflecting the specific areas of the brain that have been damaged. Common symptoms include difficulties with thinking – taking more time to process information and to form thoughts and sentences; changes in emotion and manner such as becoming low in mood, being more emotional or losing interest in things; difficulty with movement or walking leading to unsteadiness and falls; and bladder problems.

At the same time, there is a complex relationship between vascular dementia and Alzheimer's disease dementia. Many people turn out to have elements of both conditions – they will be experiencing both the degeneration of brain cells that is characteristic of Alzheimer's disease and damage to blood vessels in the brain that causes vascular dementia. This is called *'mixed' dementia*. Without a brain scan it can often be difficult for doctors to determine which condition the person has – or the relative balance of Alzheimer's disease and vascular dementia. Current evidence suggests that whilst Alzheimer's disease is the most common single form of dementia, around 50 per cent of people with dementia will have some cerebral-vascular disease, either vascular dementia or 'mixed' dementia, with both Alzheimer's disease and vascular dementia.

## Treatment and progression of vascular dementia

There is no way with our current state of knowledge that the brain damage that characterises vascular dementia can be reversed. However, it is possible that vascular dementia may be prevented, or its progression slowed down or halted, if factors that led to the underlying vascular disease are addressed. The risk of vascular disease can be significantly reduced by maintaining a healthy body weight, eating a diet that minimises saturated fats and includes lots of fruit, vegetables and fish (the 'Mediterranean diet'), drinking alcohol within safe limits, not smoking and taking regular exercise. Getting treatment for vascular-related conditions such as hypertension (high blood pressure) or diabetes will also reduce risk. If the signs and symptoms of vascular dementia do appear, adopting a healthy lifestyle and treating underlying vascular disease can slow or even stop the progression of the condition – it is possible for people to have a number of mini-strokes (TIAs) without vascular dementia developing.

Current opinion is that the AChE inhibitor drugs developed to treat Alzheimer's disease are not effective for people with vascular dementia, although they may be prescribed for those with 'mixed' dementia. If underlying vascular factors are not brought under control, vascular dementia may progress until the person experiences advanced dementia and will lead to the death of the person. As with Alzheimer's disease, this process may take some years.

## Dementia with Lewy bodies (DLB)

This is the third main type of late-onset dementia, although it is probably less common than Alzheimer's disease or vascular dementia. It is thought that approximately 5–10 per cent of people with dementia will have DLB, and recent studies suggest it is more common in men. Like Alzheimer's disease, it involves the degeneration and death of brain cells, leading to a generally gradual, progressive increase in difficulties, although memory is sometimes less affected in the early years. A person with DLB may also have periods of drowsiness or faintness and may be prone to falls, with attention and concentration sometimes fluctuating quite quickly. They may experience visual hallucinations and false perceptions when they believe they can see things that are not really there. Sleep disturbances are also quite common. Finally, the person may display signs of Parkinsonism, including stiffness of joints and tremor in the limbs that they cannot control. If the brain cells of a person with DLB are examined under a microscope, *Lewy bodies* can be seen in the areas of the brain that control movement, memory and thinking. Lewy bodies are spherical protein deposits (also found in Parkinson's disease) that form clumps and damage the way brain cells work and communicate. Some people with Parkinson's disease may develop symptoms of dementia as their disease progresses; this is known as Parkinson's disease dementia. People with DLB may also have Alzheimer's disease – also called 'mixed' dementia. A specific scan called a SPECT scan may be used to diagnose DLB, but the symptoms may be enough to make a diagnosis.

### Treatment and progression of DLB

There is at present no known way of preventing DLB and no known cure. However, the drugs used for Alzheimer's disease dementia may help with some of the symptoms of DLB, including improving thinking skills and reducing hallucinations. If AChE inhibitor drugs are prescribed, these should be given in the morning to help minimise sleep disturbance, which is a common problem in DLB. Problems with movement may respond to similar treatments used for those with Parkinson's disease such as physiotherapy and exercise, but caution is needed with the usual medication offered called Levodopa, as this can worsen hallucinations. Progression is sadly often faster than Alzheimer's disease due to the additional physical and psychological complications.

It is important to accurately diagnose DLB as some sedating drugs (called 'antipsychotic drugs') that are sometimes used to treat hallucinations in people with dementia may have particularly severe side effects if given to a person with this condition (see Chapter 8).

## TYPES OF YOUNG-ONSET DEMENTIA

We saw in Chapter 1 that around 40,000 people in the UK are diagnosed with young-onset dementia, defined as dementia that occurs before the age of 65. This figure is likely to be a substantial under-estimate – some research suggests that there may actually be double that number, with many cases undiagnosed. If recognising late-onset dementia can be difficult, identifying dementia in younger people is often considerably harder, for two main reasons. First, because of its rarity, dementia is not expected to occur in younger people, and so, if a person is appearing to think or act in unusual ways, they or their family and friends are likely to attribute their signs and symptoms to other factors, such as stress or other mental or physical disorders. Second, the early signs of several types of young-onset dementia are often not the same as those of late-onset dementias, leading again to possible misidentification. Those with young-onset dementia are more likely to be diagnosed with rarer forms of dementia and to have a genetically inherited form of dementia.

'I think there are huge difficulties for younger people with getting a diagnosis. They are often diagnosed with depression, and you can go with the tablets and a year or more goes by and nothing happens.' (Family member)

'People often don't believe you when you have young-onset dementia because symptoms are often more hidden.' (Person with dementia)

## Young-onset Alzheimer's disease dementia

Alzheimer's disease is the most common cause of young-onset dementia, accounting for around one-third of all cases of dementia in those under the age of 65. Indeed, Dr Alois Alzheimer's first published case description in 1907 of the disease that bears his name was of a woman in her early 50s. Alzheimer's disease has the same features in younger people as in those in later life, and the condition progresses in the same way. Treatments available for Alzheimer's disease dementia may also help younger people for a time. There appears to be a rare sub-type of Alzheimer's disease that affects younger people that has a strongly genetic element to it, with several members of the same family affected by the condition. If someone has a strong family history of Alzheimer's at a young age, a doctor may suggest genetic testing to close relatives and refer them on for genetic counselling.

## Other diseases that lead to young-onset dementia

The other main late-onset dementias, vascular dementia and DLB, can also occur in people under the age of 65. Many other diseases can cause dementia in younger people (whilst also occasionally appearing for the first time when the person is over 65). Almost all are progressive, and the person will eventually experience the profound difficulties of advanced dementia, but early on different types may have their own particular features. There are some specialist centres and groups in the UK for those affected by rarer dementias, and details can be found in the Resources section at the end of the book. The following are some of the more prevalent young-onset conditions.

## Fronto-temporal dementia (FTD)
## (previously known as Pick's disease)

This term covers a number of conditions and accounts for around 12 per cent of dementias in younger people. It includes four different conditions that are all degenerative and lead to the death of brain cells. Although FTD is more common in people aged between 45 and 65, it can also occur in older people. Changes begin in the frontal and temporal lobes of the cortex – at the front and on each side of the brain. These areas are mostly concerned with governing our social abilities, 'executive function', behaviour (frontal lobe) and language skills (temporal lobes), and it is these aspects that are initially affected rather than memory. Some FTDs also affect movement and balance.

'People instantly think of memory and fronto-temporal dementia isn't really about the memory; the major thing is sequencing and changes in behaviour.' (Person with dementia)

- *Behavioural variant (bvFTD):* This type of FTD, as the name suggests, mostly affects the person's manner and behaviour. Early signs can include apparent changes in the person's personality such as apathy, loss of empathy, moodiness or inexplicable lapses in social etiquette. Other features may include repetition or obsessive behaviour, sometimes including changes in eating habits plus difficulties with complex tasks. The person may become either much more subdued or more outgoing than before. Social lapses may become more prominent, with the person perhaps becoming quite rude or disinhibited.

- *Primary progressive aphasia (PPA):* This condition affects communication, including speech, understanding and writing. As memory and judgement are not usually affected initially, people may become very frustrated and depressed as a result.

- *Corticobasal degeneration (CBD):* This is a progressive condition, which initially starts with sudden problems with controlling limbs, loss of balance and coordination. As it progresses, other symptoms may include muscle spasms and stiffness, difficulties with speech and swallowing, as well as cognitive decline.

- *Progressive supra-nuclear palsy (PSP):* This affects coordination of balance and movement and primarily affects the ability to move the eyes. It is caused by progressive damage to the cells in the brain that control eye movements, and can progress to include the throat and mouth, affecting speech and swallowing. Some people may also experience changes in their behaviour, clumsiness or stiffness, and it is often confused with Parkinson's disease.

These conditions can be particularly difficult for families as the symptoms are often more unusual, more challenging to cope with and there is often less support available. It is important with behavioural lapses that others realise that the person 'can't help it' – it is purely an effect of the disease process.

## Huntington's disease

This is a disease that affects the areas of the brain that govern thinking and also parts of the brain that regulate the motor nerves that control the action of muscles. This means that the person has progressive difficulties in movement and the use of muscles as well as developing dementia. Huntington's disease is caused by a single dominant gene, which means that a child of a person with the condition has a 50 per cent chance of developing the illness themselves. The first signs of the condition usually appear when the person is in their 30s. The person will develop 'tics' or involuntary muscular movements, and their personality may start to change, becoming moody and sometimes uncontrollably aggressive. Cognitive difficulties include issues with short-term memory and concentration.

As the disease progresses, the person experiences increasing problems with involuntary movements and also weight loss. Cognitive difficulties also increase, and the person can be particularly prone to mood swings, depression and stubbornness. As time goes on, the dementia becomes more advanced. People can live with Huntington's disease for 10–20 years.

### Alcohol-related dementia

Alcohol can lead to dementia in more than one way. It is a toxin that can damage brain cells, and excessive consumption over many years can sometimes cause enough damage to lead to dementia (this condition is called *alcoholic dementia*). More commonly, people who misuse alcohol risk developing *Korsakoff's syndrome*, a dementia-like condition that results from a deficiency in vitamin B1 (thiamine). This is thought to account for about 10 per cent of dementias in younger people. Although Korsakoff's syndrome is most commonly associated with alcohol abuse, it can also be caused by excessive vomiting in pregnancy and bulimia (an eating disorder). People can become deficient in thiamine because their diet does not give them the right nutrients. Excessive alcohol consumption interferes with the body's ability to effectively use thiamine as well as the liver's ability to store vitamins. Symptoms usually start with memory loss but can also include changes in manner or behaviour, and difficulty in acquiring new information or skills.

In its early stages, the condition is known as *Wernicke encephalopathy*. If the underlying vitamin deficiency is identified and treated with high doses of thiamine at an early stage, the symptoms can be reversed. If not, the person often goes on to develop Korsakoff's syndrome. Unfortunately the lifestyles of those who excessively misuse alcohol often prevent them from accessing such medical attention, and their difficulties can become permanent.

All in all, moderating our alcohol consumption is an important step in reducing our risk of developing dementia. Although few of us drink heavily or recklessly enough to develop alcohol-related dementia, as we have seen, drinking above safe limits increases the risk for all of us of vascular disease, which, in turn, is a strong factor in the development of both vascular dementia and Alzheimer's disease.

### Posterior-cortical atrophy (PCA)

This condition is sometimes called 'Benson's syndrome' and is caused by degeneration of the brain cells at the back (posterior) of the brain, which helps us make sense of what we are seeing. Readers may be familiar with the author Terry Pratchett who was affected by this type of dementia. Although he has sadly now died, he continued to work with support and campaigned about dementia for a number of years after his diagnosis. The damage is similar to Alzheimer's disease but the effects are different due to where the damage occurs. Early symptoms include difficulties with vision and perception rather than memory, and people may have problems with reading, judging distances, recognising objects, light sensitivity, thinking skills and coordination. As the condition progresses, memory, language and problem-solving will also start to deteriorate. The same treatments given to those with Alzheimer's disease dementia may also help people with PCA.

### Neurological diseases that may include dementia amongst their symptoms

A number of conditions that are usually grouped within neurology may, in their late phases, lead to dementia-like symptoms as well as to increasing physical disability. These include Parkinson's disease, multiple sclerosis and muscular dystrophy, amongst others. Dementia may also occur in the late phase of AIDS, although, in Western countries at least, new drug treatments have improved the life expectancy of those with HIV infection and reduced the extent of AIDS- or HIV-related dementia.

## DELIRIUM – AN ADDITIONAL NOTE

Although delirium is not a type of dementia, it needs a special mention as it is so commonly misdiagnosed as dementia and can cause significant problems for those with dementia.

It is recognised by a sudden change in the person's mental state, which usually fluctuates and can include increased confusion, disorientation or difficulty with concentration. There are two types of delirium – *hyperactive delirium* or *hypoactive delirium*. Hyperactive delirium is when people may become very restless, confused, agitated or distressed and their speech may be confused or rambling. Sleep is often disturbed and some people experience hallucinations (seeing things that are not there) or delusions (believing things that are not true). In hypoactive delirium people may become more sleepy or withdrawn. This is harder to spot, particularly when the person is in more advanced stages of dementia. Whilst some of these symptoms are seen in dementia, delirium is different in that it has a sudden onset and symptoms fluctuate. It is caused by a number of factors such as infections, pain or dehydration, which are all treatable. Older people and people with dementia are at increased risk of developing delirium, and those with repeated episodes of delirium seem to be more at risk of going on to develop dementia and have a higher risk of dying.

It is essential that delirium is diagnosed early to find out the cause and that this is treated to prevent further deterioration. With the right treatment, symptoms should ease after a few days, but this may take much longer for people with dementia. Delirium can be very distressing, both for the person and their family, and simple communication strategies such as those described in Chapter 6 may be useful in supporting the person.

# CHAPTER 4

# Sources of Support for People with Dementia and their Families and Friends

The focus of this book is to assist family members and friends to support and care for a person with dementia. However, families and friends should not undertake this responsibility unaided. We have already discussed the importance of supporting each other in Chapter 2, and in this chapter we give an overview of other sources of support available in the UK, including health and social care professionals and lay and peer support. We also introduce some of the financial support that may be available from the UK government.

## PROFESSIONAL HEALTH SERVICES

It is quite hard to generalise about professional health and social care services that may be helpful to people with dementia and their families. A number of factors may influence a person accessing services:

- Some services may be more or less appropriate at different times.

- Services may be configured differently in different parts of the country and some may be less available in places.

- Some services are specific to people with dementia, whilst the person may access others due to other physical or mental health needs that they may have along with dementia.

- Whilst health care is free at the point of access, many social care services are means-tested and access may be related to the person's ability to pay for them.

## Doctors

We saw in the last chapter that the person's *general practitioner (GP)* is the first port of call for getting an assessment and diagnosis of dementia, and the GP is likely to remain the focus for coordinating or providing health care. The GP may refer the person for specialised assessment and treatment from a *psychiatrist* or *neurologist*, depending on the type of dementia that the person has and the effects that the condition has on the person. Older people may have a range of co-existing physical health issues and the GP may refer to appropriate specialists. These may or may not be sensitive to the needs of people with dementia, and family members may have an important role in advocating for the person during consultations.

## Nurses

There is a range of community nursing services. These include *community mental health nurses (CMHNs)*, who provide support and advice to people with dementia living in the community and their carers. In some parts of the country *Admiral Nurses* are available. These are registered nurses who specialise in working with families affected by dementia and are supported by the charity Dementia UK (see the Resources section at the end of the book). They are often based in the community but are also available in some general hospitals, care homes and hospices. A national helpline is also available staffed by Admiral Nurses to offer support and advice when local services are not available. Other specialist dementia nurses may be available in memory services or other settings, and the person may also be referred to other *community nurses*, particularly if they have co-existing physical health issues.

## Other health care professionals

Referral to other specialist professionals may be appropriate in some cases:

- *Psychologists* provide more specialised assessment and support, including cognitive therapies for both people with dementia and family carers (see Chapter 5, page 139). Psychologists may also assist if the person has other mental health issues such as depression or anxiety.

- *Occupational therapists* can offer advice and sometimes aids to help the person live independently. They may also provide *cognitive rehabilitation*, which involves identifying goals that focus on improving or maintaining functioning in everyday life.

- *Speech and language therapists* can assist with communication issues or may be asked to provide an assessment and advice if the person has swallowing problems.

- *Dieticians* offer help with eating and concerns about nutrition. This may be as a result of dementia or another condition.

- *Continence advisors* will offer advice about managing problems with bladder or bowel control, and can advise about appropriate continence aids.

'We rely on psychosocial support from professionals including the consultant, psychiatrist, the psychologist and the Admiral Nurse. I also get support from the people I have met as a result of dementia.' (Person with dementia)

## PROFESSIONAL SOCIAL CARE SERVICES
### Social workers

Social workers are employed by local authority social services departments and will assess the person's care needs and what kinds of support they might require. They will also determine whether or how much the person will have to pay for services. Even if the person is not eligible for financial support, the *care needs assessment* is still useful, as it can provide valuable information on what services and support are relevant and available locally. The person's GP or other health or social care professionals can arrange a care needs assessment or carers can approach their local authority to request an assessment.

Carers should also be offered a *carer's assessment*. This is carried out by social workers and it is important that you ask for this, as a carer's needs are not always recognised. Assessment includes looking at the impact that caring for a person with dementia is having on you, and will then identify the type and level of support that you need to be able to carry out your role as a carer. This should result in a *support plan* which identifies what support you might need, such as respite care for the person with dementia, so that you have some time to yourself; aids, adaptations or training in how to support the person with dementia move around; or some help coming into your home. This will also include a financial assessment, and if you are eligible for support, this can be provided by direct payments to the service providing support or via a personal budget so you can pay for services yourself.

### Social care services

The local authority may directly provide such services, but it is more likely that they will be commissioned from independent or voluntary sector providers. As suggested above, some services may be more appropriate at particular times, or may suit some people more than others. Some of the types of support are explained further below.

## Day care services or centres

As the name suggests, these are facilities that people with dementia can attend during the working day whilst family members have a rest or go to work, and where they can take part in activities and socialise with others. Some day care services also invite family members to attend alongside the person with dementia, and can provide separate support for the person who is caring. Many family members find the respite that day care centres provide invaluable, and many people with dementia enjoy attending them. However, not all people with dementia relish attending day centres – if the person has, throughout their life, been reserved and private, they may not find being with other people easy. The best day centres have a wide range of activities, and staff who understand the needs of those who attend and offer advice and support to family members.

'They have offered my grandma the chance to go to community centres and things but she's not a joiner-in, she never has been, and we couldn't expect her to do it now.' (Family member)

'My husband attends a day centre two days per week and this allows me to have some time for myself and to keep on top of things. It also gives him some independence and space away from me...a little bit of life outside of my control.' (Family member)

## Activity or social groups

An increasing number and variety of groups are available, offering activities or a social setting where people with dementia and carers can meet with others with similar interests. These range from groups offering singing, music, arts and crafts, exercise or other interests, and are mostly supported by voluntary sector organisations but may be funded by health or social care. Some groups offer support for specific communities or seldom-heard groups. These groups are often highly valued as they can support individual preferences or lifestyles and help maintain activity, social engagement and well-being. At the same time, support groups are not to everyone's taste, and some people may have practical problems with attending meetings.

## Dementia cafes or meeting centres

These may be similar to the less formal activity or social groups described above, but are usually organised by local memory services, or specialist statutory or voluntary sector dementia services. They offer a space where people with dementia and family carers can meet others. They may include speakers or therapy-based support.

## Home care

If the person has been assessed as requiring assistance with aspects of their physical health or daily living care, care at home can be provided to help the person with such things as getting bathed and dressed or at mealtimes. Provision of home care can be very variable, with some authorities offering more than others, and the extent that people with dementia have to pay for such care may also vary from area to area. Whilst many home carers are skilled and committed, the quality of home care has been criticised, with complaints that visits are extremely brief, staff given strict limits on how long they should spend with a person and often a lack of consistency of staff, with different workers attending each day so that no one actually gets to know the person with dementia.

'We've had some really lovely carers who genuinely do really nice things for my grandma and that really helps...it's nice when you can feel you can trust people.' (Family member)

'Introducing a home carer was very difficult as my wife didn't want any help; the first person didn't work as my wife didn't like her. However, when Jenny started, it worked well from the beginning. She was very skilled and did things like going shopping with my wife, made her feel included. This was such a relief. It took a few weeks before they settled in but eventually my wife thought Jenny was lovely.' (Family member)

## Personal assistants and private carers

Sometimes families directly employ people to provide care, and the state may provide a personalised care budget that the family can spend as they wish. They may employ professional carers from an agency, which helps to ensure liability and protection, or some people may choose to employ a friend or neighbour directly to offer care. There can be great advantages in being able to choose the right person and in ensuring continuity of carers, but it is also important that advice is sought about how to protect the person receiving care, who may be vulnerable. In addition, managing a budget can also be difficult for people in the early phases of dementia or family members, so this should be thought through carefully.

'I have discussed the future with my wife, and we both want me to remain at home as long as is possible. We would rather buy in care than pay care home fees. I love where I live and it is a very suitable home for someone with advanced dementia.' (Person with dementia)

'I arranged for one day a week replacement care at home to give me a break, and sometimes I had a stretch of five consecutive days. It was always the same person who was employed to come in. Without those breaks I don't think I could have made it.' (Family member)

## 24-hour respite care

Other forms of respite care than day or home care may be available to enable the person's main carer to take a break. Sometimes it can be arranged for someone to stay with the person with dementia whilst the main carer goes away for a holiday – other family members or friends may, of course, take on this role, or a paid carer may be employed. Alternatively, a person with dementia may themselves spend a week or two in a care home whilst their carer has a break. Again, paying for respite care may be an issue, and the change of environment as well as quality of care are important considerations.

## LAY AND PEER SUPPORT SERVICES

Many carers and people with dementia find having a network of informal lay or peer support invaluable. The growth of dementia-friendly community initiatives and groups, some of which are supported by national voluntary sector organisations, can be a lifeline for people.

### Peer support groups

Groups of family members and friends of people with dementia may come together, often facilitated by voluntary sector organisations, in order to meet each other, share experiences and help each other out. Some peer support groups have separate get-togethers for people with dementia themselves whilst their carers are having their own meetings. As with dementia cafes, invited speakers may attend to give talks on important topics. Some such groups and organisations have also been instrumental in giving a voice to people with dementia and family carers in influencing policy such as:

- tide (together in dementia everyday) for family carers

- DEEP (Dementia Engagement & Empowerment Project) groups for people with dementia.

Information about these can be found in the Resources section at the end of the book.

### Internet-based support

The growth of internet-based and social media platforms may fill the gap in some cases and help connect people who are sharing similar experiences. A word of caution, though, when scouring the internet for support is to check the background and locality of the source, as sometimes information can be out of date or inaccurate. Some recommended sources are offered in the Resources section.

'I get most support from people living with dementia who I meet, either in a DEEP group or when we go to conferences and meetings. We chat, we laugh, we can say things we cannot tell our other halves.' (Person with dementia)

'Self-help and peer support have been crucial for both my husband and myself. Finding peers and making a difference by doing what we can, whilst we can, has kept us going.' (Family member)

## HOUSING OPTIONS

There is a range of housing options to consider as people need more help, and it is useful to have conversations with the person you are supporting about their preferences for the future as early as possible. Whilst needs may change as the condition progresses, at least the conversation will help guide and inform decisions as they arise.

### Supported accommodation

As a compromise between living alone and entering residential care, some people with dementia live in 'supported accommodation'. This may include sheltered or retirement homes, where the person has their own flat or apartment, and lives more or less independently. Support may be arranged via social services or private agencies or may be available on site for some or all of the day. Alternatively, 'assisted living' and 'extra care schemes' provide a more intensive level of support than traditional sheltered housing. There will usually be at least one member of staff on hand 24 hours a day.

Additional facilities are often available for people who are not able to get out regularly, perhaps including a restaurant, shop, gym, hobby room, and so on. Activities may be arranged regularly, as in sheltered housing, commonly with an emphasis on improving or maintaining residents' health and well-being.

Another new development is that of 'care villages' in which a number of different types of accommodation are available designed to support people as their needs change. An initiative from the Netherlands, in which the environment has been designed specifically to enable people with dementia to remain as independent as possible, has received great interest, and a number of similar dementia villages are being established in the UK.

As dementia progresses, a move to a *care home* may be considered. We will consider the issues around residential care in Chapter 9.

## ADVICE AND SIGNPOSTING SERVICES

In some areas steps are being taken to set up services that people with early dementia and their families may contact for advice and signposting to other sources of professional help. Advice services have links to health and social services and can make it easier for families to access such services if difficulties arise.

### Telephone support services

Both Dementia UK and the Alzheimer's Society have helplines that can offer advice and support to all who contact them. The Admiral Nurse Dementia Helpline, supported by Dementia UK, is staffed by experienced dementia specialist nurses who can offer skilled emotional support and advice about more complex issues. Telephone numbers are included in the Resources section.

## Internet sites

Charities and other bodies have extensive websites packed with information and advice. These often also include forums or chatrooms where those supporting a person with dementia – and sometimes people with dementia themselves – can communicate online with others.

'I recently used the Alzheimer's Society Talking Point and it was useful to find out how other people cope with difficult situations; it was quite reassuring.' (Family member)

## SUPPORT SERVICES ARE THERE TO HELP!

Many carers of people with dementia feel it is their responsibility alone to look after the person, and may feel guilt or a sense of weakness when considering accessing support. Our advice to you is clear: don't feel you have to carry all of the load yourself! Use your GP, local social services department and other local sources to find out what is available in your area, and don't be afraid to be assertive at getting appropriate support. The alternative is that you may exhaust yourself, and the person with dementia may have a reduced quality of life.

## FINANCIAL HELP AND BENEFITS

A benefit is a sum of money given to a person by the government to help them meet their day-to-day living needs. It may be that some readers are already receiving benefits of one kind or another (the most obvious one being the state pension), but others may have never applied for or been given any government benefit. The benefits system in the UK is bewilderingly complex and subject to change, and as such it is beyond the scope of this book to guide readers through all the possible benefits that may be available to the person with dementia or their carers. We can, however, provide an overview of what might be accessible, and encourage you to explore further and to apply for benefits for which you may be eligible. Research has shown that caring for a person with dementia can place a considerable financial burden on the family, and it is in their best interests to access whatever financial support is available.

## Basic principles of the UK benefits system

As suggested above, the benefits system is not simple:

- There are no benefits that exclusively apply to people with dementia or their carers. Families must determine what they are eligible for out of a range of more generalised benefits.

- Many benefits require an assessment of need carried out by a professional, and are only awarded if set criteria are met.

- Some benefits are paid directly to the person with dementia (although they may be accessed by family members who have power of attorney – see Chapter 5), whilst others are paid to the person's carer.

- Some benefits are given to all regardless of income, whilst others are means-tested.

- Some are given at a flat rate, whilst others have different rates according to assessed need.

- Different benefits originate from different government services and will have to be applied for separately.

- Some benefits apply to 'working-age' adults, whilst others apply to older people.

- Receiving a benefit may affect entitlement to another benefit – sometimes increasing eligibility and sometimes reducing it.

- Benefits are in a continuous state of flux, and some benefits formerly awarded are being replaced by newer versions.

- The benefits system is in some ways different in Scotland and Northern Ireland compared with England and Wales.

Confused? So are we! To add to the complexity, there is no single government agency or professional who can tell a family exactly what they are entitled to. You can try the online Benefits Calculator, which will help to advise you on what financial help is available.[1] Some third sector organisations offer a benefits advice service, and we would urge readers to consider accessing such services.

These are the most relevant benefits that are potentially available to people with dementia and their carers, although readers may be entitled to other benefits, depending on income, age and circumstances (correct at the time of writing):

- *Attendance Allowance* is available to people over 65 years old in the UK if their ability to keep safe or look after their own personal care is affected by physical or mental illness, or disability. Claiming Attendance Allowance will not reduce any other income received and it is tax-free. It is awarded at either a lower or higher rate according to assessed needs. Those awarded it may become entitled to other benefits, such as Pension Credit, Housing Benefit or Council Tax Reduction, or an increase in these.

- *Carer's Allowance* is paid to the carer of someone who receives other benefits, like Attendance Allowance or a Personal Independence Payment. Claimees need to be 16 or over, spend at least 35 hours a week caring for someone, earn no more than £110 a week, and not be receiving some other benefits, such as Incapacity Benefit or a state pension. The person being cared for may lose some of their benefits if their carer receives this allowance, so it's important to get advice before making a claim.

---

1   www.gov.uk/benefits-adviser

- *Carer's Credit* is a benefit paid by the UK government to carers that helps build the carer's entitlement to the basic and additional State Pension. Your income, savings or investments won't affect eligibility for Carer's Credit, but you need to be caring for someone for at least 20 hours a week, be over 16 but under State Pension age, and be looking after someone who gets specific benefits, like Attendance Allowance.

- *Personal Independence Payment (PIP)* is a benefit that helps with some of the extra costs caused by long-term ill health or a disability. Claimees need to be aged 16 to 64 and living in the UK. PIP is tax-free and you can get it whether you're in or out of work.

- *Council Tax Reduction* is applied to a person with dementia who receives either Attendance Allowance or PIP at a certain rate. Sometimes carers are not counted for Council Tax if they are living with and caring for a person with dementia who gets the higher rate of Attendance Allowance or PIP.

- *Direct Payments (cash)* may be made by local authority social services departments to people who need community care services. This allows the person (or their legal representatives) to choose and buy the services they need instead of getting them from their local council. The payment is means-tested following an assessment from the local authority, and it should be enough to cover the support that the person with dementia has been assessed as needing.

- *NHS Continuing Healthcare.* Some people with long-term complex health needs qualify for free social care arranged and funded solely by the NHS. NHS Continuing Healthcare can be provided in a variety of settings outside hospital, such as in the person's own home or in a care home.

The application process for these benefits can be long-winded and involves making a clear case for why the person meets the criteria. Accessing advice from organisations that provide such a service is highly recommended. So is perseverance – readers owe it to themselves and the person they are supporting to get the financial help from the government that they are entitled to.

'We use our direct payments to fund our travel and campsites for our motor home which has been invaluable for maintaining well-being and mood for both of us.' (Family member)

# Understanding Dementia as it Progresses

PART 2

# Understanding Dementia as it Progresses

# CHAPTER 5

# The Early Years of Dementia

'I may have dementia but dementia doesn't have me.' (Person with dementia)

## THE CHARACTERISTICS OF EARLY DEMENTIA

As discussed in Chapter 3, it can be difficult to identify and diagnose dementia precisely, as early changes or difficulties are sometimes attributed to 'normal' ageing or other health problems. Also, each person will be different in the way they experience and react to early symptoms. This will depend on the type of dementia they have, their individual coping strategies, their general health and their social situation. However, a person with early dementia is likely to have some characteristic symptoms. Alzheimer's Research UK has a helpful list of the most common difficulties of early dementia. Initially these are likely to include one or more of the following:

- Forgetting recent events, names and faces
- Asking the same things, often in a short space of time
- Putting things in the wrong place
- Finding it hard to pay attention or make simple decisions
- Not being sure about the date or time of day
- Getting lost, mostly in places that are new

- Finding it hard to use the right words or understand other people's words

- Changes in how someone feels, like becoming sad or easily upset or losing interest in things.

These difficulties can cause real problems with managing daily life. For a younger person, problems experienced with planning, organising and carrying out complex tasks will compromise their ability to work. For a retired person, such 'executive function' difficulties will make it harder to carry out usual activities, such as hobbies, childcare or voluntary work. Increasing forgetfulness will also affect the person's daily life if they forget appointments or neglect important obligations such as paying bills. Family members and friends may well notice the person's mood and behaviour in social situations changing, with the person perhaps becoming distant and withdrawn, finding it harder to contribute to conversation or activities.

'We had always been fairly equal in our relationship but I began to notice changes in my husband's behaviour, like not sharing responsibilities in the house, housework, cooking.' (Family member)

'Frustration is probably the most accurate word to describe what living with dementia is like. I get frustrated when I can't manage the things I used to do.' (Person with dementia)

Despite this, the person will usually still be able to remain independent, and keep active. Participation in social interaction and activities remains important and should still be possible. Even activities such as driving are not impossible in early dementia. Also, the person will often retain awareness of their situation and will still be able to contribute to family discussions and to decisions about their future living and care arrangements. It is important for all of us to have a sense of control and independence, and this may be felt even more by people with early dementia, who rightly want to maintain their abilities. In fact, doing so can contribute significantly to the person's well-being and help maintain function.

> 'As long as I keep myself organised with my iPad and iPhone and take time to regularly check these, I can manage my life okay.' (Person with dementia)

However, the person may need the assistance and support of family and friends in order to maintain aspects of their usual lifestyle for as long as possible. In the rest of this chapter we examine how family members and friends can help a person with early dementia, and how they can maintain their usual relationships with the person.

## EMPATHY AND EARLY DEMENTIA

Many of us have some long-standing cognitive 'difficulties' that can mirror aspects of early dementia:

- Jane has a chronically poor memory. She regards herself and is regarded by others as 'absent-minded' and frequently forgets appointments or fails to recognise people she has met before.

- Charles has a very poor sense of direction. He finds it hard to understand maps and often loses his way when driving to unfamiliar places.

- Saleema finds it hard to take in complex information. She struggles to understand bureaucratic processes and often fills in official forms wrongly.

- Robert finds it hard to make difficult decisions. He feels overwhelmed with the various conflicting facts and opinions that he is bombarded with on the matter in question, and 'can't see the wood for the trees'.

- Kelly finds interacting with her physical environment hard. She struggles to understand how things relate to each other or fit together. If she tries to carry out such things as do-it-yourself (DIY) activities or decorating, they often go horribly wrong.

- Mohammed finds reading and writing hard, and has recently been diagnosed with dyslexia.

Few of us understand the world around us perfectly, or feel completely confident in responding appropriately to all the demands the world places on us. As discussed in Chapter 3, none of these things are themselves diagnostic of dementia; they simply reflect normal human variability. We would only become concerned and suspect dementia if we perceived a significant unexplained change in our cognitive abilities – a noticeable decline in ability from whatever level we were accustomed to.

We can, however, draw on our own experiences when considering how we might empathise with and support a person with early dementia. How do we feel about our own cognitive shortcomings? Perhaps we laugh them off or even exaggerate them for effect. On the other hand, we may be more or less distressed and angry with ourselves and regard our difficulties as signs of weakness. Perhaps we will deny that there are things that we aren't good at and put huge efforts into trying to do those things, every failure making us more determined to try again. People with early dementia may react to their own growing difficulties in any of these ways.

> 'Sometimes I wear a mask to help me cope with my difficulties, but I need people to empathise and step into my shoes. They need to watch, to think about what I'm saying and not to take what is on the surface.' (Person with dementia)

How do we compensate for those cognitive difficulties we ourselves experience? Some of us have found strategies for helping us do things we find hard. The forgetful person has learnt to write down reminders, set alarms and keep lists of things they have to do. When meeting a person in the street they don't immediately recognise, they may use basic social skills to interact with the person whilst pretending that they know who they are talking to. The person with a poor sense of direction writes themselves clear instructions for their journey before setting out or uses a navigation app. Someone with dyslexia may have acquired aids to reading and writing such as large print books and word processors to avoid having to handwrite.

In other cases we seek the advice or assistance of others. The person faced with a complex bureaucratic form may go through it with a friend who has completed the same form previously. The person faced with a complicated decision may talk it through with family, or consult a counsellor. The clumsy person will enlist the help of someone more competent to assist with carrying out a DIY task. Ultimately, of course, we may decide that the thing we are struggling with is too hard for us and we decide to either not bother with it or ask someone else to do it for us, as a favour or in a paid capacity.

Again, people with early dementia will employ any or all of these strategies when managing their own difficulties. In some cases it is possible for the person to continue to do things themselves by modifying their way of doing them, sometimes with the assistance of technology. In other cases the person may still be able to contribute towards getting things done, but will need the help of others in order to successfully fulfil the task.

'I don't feel safe because of my dementia due to my orientation. I need people to know that I am not safe on the roads and they need to look out for me.' (Person with dementia)

However, some activities, due to specific changes in the brain, may present significant difficulty. In these cases it may be best for the person to give up certain activities and allow others to support them or take them over. These can be difficult decisions, especially if the person is giving up something they value, or lacks awareness that they are not able to perform as they used to.

For family members and friends, the aim is to offer just enough help to enable the person with dementia to live their life successfully and safely without taking away the person's independence unnecessarily. Achieving this balance can clearly be hard. How do we know that a person is unable to do something unless they try to do it? But what if they attempt an activity, find they are unable to do it and come to harm as a result? Also, the person's ability to be independent will depend on the nature of the activity – they may be able to carry out some activities without any problem but may struggle with others. Equally, the person's abilities will change over time. Family members and friends need to know the person very well in order to judge when to give help or when to allow the person to continue to do things for themselves – and sometimes they have to cross their fingers and hope for the best.

## AWARENESS AND CAPACITY IN EARLY DEMENTIA

We discussed in Chapter 1 the idea of awareness in dementia and have suggested that often people with early dementia retain considerable awareness, both of the world around them and of their own difficulties. This is an appropriate time to introduce a related concept, that of *capacity* (also known as 'mental capacity' or 'legal capacity'). This is a legal term that governs both what decisions people with dementia are able to make for themselves in a legal sense and when others, particularly family members and friends, can legally step in and make decisions on their behalf. Capacity is also a useful concept in assisting us with empathising with people with early dementia as it is closely linked to the idea of awareness, and it can help us decide what level of support the person may need at a given time with specific activities.

### The concept of capacity

Capacity means possessing the ability to perceive and understand the world accurately, and to respond to events and circumstances and make decisions in a considered and appropriate way. In short, a person who has capacity 'knows what they are doing' – however they are behaving, they are doing so with an understanding of the situation and having consciously decided to act in that way. It may be that in some cases others would not act in that way or would not have made that decision and may find the person's behaviour strange, but if the person knows what they are doing…they have capacity.

In the UK the legal criteria for judging whether a person has the capacity to make a decision are that the person must be able to:

- Understand information given to them about a particular decision

- Retain that information long enough to be able to make the decision

- Weigh up the information available to make the decision

- Communicate the decision.

Some people will lack capacity (this is sometimes called *incapacity*). It is not just people with dementia who may lack capacity; members of other groups including people with learning disabilities, people with acquired brain injury and some people with mental and physical health problems may also lack capacity in the legal sense. Capacity is not a global concept but it is specific to situations and times, so a person may lack capacity related to some aspects of their life but not to others, or may lack capacity at a certain time (for example, when acutely mentally ill) and may regain capacity in the future.

The capacity of people with dementia to make decisions will be compromised as dementia damages cognitive abilities. However, it must not be assumed that all people with dementia lack capacity in the legal sense – many people with early dementia will meet the legal criteria at least some of the time. This has important implications for family members and friends of a person with dementia, not just in ensuring they keep within the law, but also because it enshrines a fundamental ethical stance. We should presume that the person retains capacity to make their own decisions unless it is clear that they cannot. We should do what we can to help the person make their own decisions, or contribute to those decisions, if it is possible for them to do so. Even if their decision is not one we would prefer them to make, we must not assume that it results from a lack of capacity. Finally, if it is decided that the person does lack capacity and that others should make decisions for them, then those decisions must be made in the person's best interests, maintaining as much independence for the person as possible.

Hopefully we can see how the concepts of mental capacity and awareness are linked – although again, we should not regard them as one and the same. However, we can certainly say that the more the person appears to retain awareness of their world and their condition, the more likely they are to retain the capacity to make decisions – even if family members and friends don't always agree with the decisions the person makes.

'There are judgements sometimes made about what people with dementia can or cannot do or want to see or hear or do – these should be challenged.' (Person with dementia)

## MAINTAINING RELATIONSHIPS AND KEEPING ACTIVE IN EARLY DEMENTIA

As we saw in Chapter 2, maintaining relationships, keeping active and social inclusion are important in supporting someone's well-being. People with early dementia can usually continue with the relationships and friendships that they already have and continue to carry out many of their accustomed leisure activities, especially if they retain a level of awareness. At the same time, family members and friends will need to adapt to the person's developing difficulties if this is to happen. It is important for the continued well-being of a person with early dementia that family members and friends understand and apply three broad principles, as shown in the figure below.

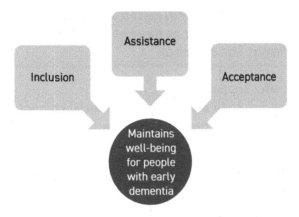

It is important that efforts are made to *include* the person in social and leisure activities. The person may well need to be *assisted* to carry out their accustomed activities, or to partake in social occasions. Finally, family members and friends may need to display a measure of *acceptance* if the person's difficulties lead to them experiencing problems in social situations or in carrying out activities. We now consider these principles in more detail.

## Inclusion

People with dementia need to maintain social relationships, carry out activities and be actively included. This does not always happen. Sadly research has shown that people with dementia can often become 'socially excluded', leading to isolation, impoverished lives and perhaps swifter progression of their condition. Friends and even family members may avoid social contact with the person, through awkwardness, lack of understanding of how to interact with the person or concern regarding the contrast between how the person is now compared with how they used to be. Stigma and prejudice within society can reinforce these socially excluding attitudes.

'Other people have been the main challenge, especially at the beginning.' (Person with dementia)

> 'My non-dementia friends don't really understand or want to talk about my disease, as they just don't really believe I have it.' (Person with dementia)

## How to offer support

Inclusion has both a practical and a social component, but these are closely interlinked. The simple fact is that for a person with dementia to feel socially included they have to *be* socially included – family members and friends must make the effort to include the person in what they are doing, and help the person to continue with their accustomed activities. The person should continue to receive invitations to social events, and family and friends must accept invitations from the person. The person should be supported and encouraged to still do activities or to be part of clubs and societies. Many people with early dementia get immense support from meeting others who have dementia, such as at the DEEP groups across England (see Chapter 4). Many people with early dementia will have retired from full-time employment, but some may still be at work and will want to continue. Increasingly, employers are being required to make what are called 'reasonable adjustments' to enable someone to carry on working. If the person wishes to continue to work and is able to do so with support or in a different role, then understanding their rights and challenging efforts to force them to leave their job is an important consideration.

> 'I have kept involved in doing as many of the things I can such as playing my music. A lot of these things can be done, as long as you've got people who are aware of your diagnosis and are checking to make sure you don't do something daft.' (Person with dementia)

> 'My husband's diagnosis was devastating for our future plans but I was keen to keep life as normal as possible. I have always needed to go out and made sure we still did this as much as possible.' (Family member)

The role of friends is crucial in ensuring that a person with early dementia continues to feel included. As stated above, friends often drift away from the person, or leave the responsibility of supporting the person to family members. We can sometimes be 'easy come, easy go' when it comes to friendships and social relationships. However, as the saying goes, 'a friend in need is a friend indeed', and few are needier than people with dementia.

'As time has gone on it's made lot of difference to social relations. We have a lot of friends who don't find it easy especially as my husband's behaviour has become more difficult. Other friends have become closer and offer to sit with my husband and that's really important. Some friends and neighbours have drifted away.' (Family member)

People with dementia may well need practical help in remaining socially included. This can be as simple as having someone collect them and take them home again if they are no longer able to drive. Again, family members and friends may need to make some effort to involve the person in family and social life.

## Assistance

As well as practical assistance with getting to and from social events and activities, people with early dementia may also need assistance from others with actually participating in those events and activities, due to the cognitive difficulties they are experiencing. If this is the case, family members and friends need to use empathy. If a person with dementia is experiencing difficulty with participating or socialising, endeavour to understand where the person has problems and try and find ways of compensating. As pointed out in Chapter 1, difficulties may arise with the person's understanding of the world around them, or with the person's ability to respond appropriately to events in their world.

## How to offer support

For many, a feature of early dementia is likely to be memory loss, the person in particular having difficulty remembering new information, but also sometimes forgetting things that they would have previously remembered as a matter of routine, such as paying a bill on time or taking their key with them when going out. Sometimes the person might forget where they are when away from their home and may not be able to find their way home. Family members and friends can assist the person by providing memory aids. These might include drawing up lists of things the person must remember to do, phoning or texting them with reminders of appointments, or drawing clear directions to help the person get about. It should be anticipated that the person might not remember things said to them, and we should be prepared to repeat ourselves, or write down important messages. Mobile phones can be valuable aids that family and friends can use to send the person reminders and as a source of help in emergencies. There are an increasing number of assistive technology devices that can help support someone's independence (see below).

If someone has memory difficulties, this will clearly affect their ability to respond to events. It may be as simple as the person not remembering the name of someone who is talking to them, or forgetting an appointment. The person may forget to take important medicines. Again, tactful reminders are helpful and will be appreciated by the person.

The person may begin to experience difficulties with maintaining attention and carrying out complex tasks (executive function). This may lead to the person struggling to keep up with others in conversations or when taking part in some activities or hobbies. Family members and friends may assist by recognising where the person has problems and offering guidance and, if possible, making the activity simpler. It is easy to overestimate the cognitive abilities of a person with early dementia as the person is likely to retain superficial social skills, so the person may put on a 'good front' and conceal the fact that they are struggling to understand or keep up with what is going on.

'When giving me choices, it's much easier to see the choices, photos, food items, clothing, etc., rather than rely on my mind and memory, otherwise my stock answer is usually "no".' (Person with dementia)

If the person was used to taking part in more complex activities, it may be the case that these become too hard for the person to follow, and family and friends may need to tactfully suggest to the person that they might find it more satisfying to take up something less demanding. The person may need to be assisted with making the switch to another activity. For example, a person who was an enthusiastic member of a classical choir may find it increasingly hard to learn complex pieces, but may enjoy singing in a community choir.

Language and communication difficulties may also start to emerge. At this point the person is likely to retain the ability to understand language and will know what others are saying to them, but their ability to respond appropriately may start to be compromised, the person in particular finding it hard to find the names of things and sometimes muddling up sentences. Patience is required on the part of those conversing with the person. We may need to give the person extra time to get their message across or to tactfully ask the person to repeat the message.

Another thing that can try the patience of families and friends is the tendency for some people with early dementia to become very repetitive in what they say, sometimes repeating the same thing many times in a conversation or including the same messages in each conversation they have. We must realise that this comes from the person's memory difficulties, the person forgetting that they have said the same thing before (we will discuss these matters further in Chapter 6).

We may also notice the person's manner or behaviour starting to change – as discussed in Chapter 3, this is often the first sign of behavioural variant fronto-temporal dementia. Sometimes the person may become more touchy, anxious, rude or even aggressive, and family and friends must adopt a calm and un-provoking manner. Tact and skilful communication will help resolve potentially problematic situations.

> 'One of the daft arguments we have with grandma is about getting her to the hairdressers; my mum's very keen that she keeps up with that, so we take her every week. Sometimes when we go round, for no reason at all she'll shout "I'm not going" and that's not the grandma I remember. I tend to make a joke of it where I can – one thing grandma is good at talking about is the weather, we have a lot of conversations about the weather and normally over and over again, so I say to her, "Next week it might be raining and we might not want to go then, so we really should go this week."' (Family member)

The person may appear more vacant or detached than before, and sometimes may appear rather self-absorbed and less interested in other people. This is a sign that their ability to understand and manage all the complexities of their social world is starting to become impaired, their memory and attention difficulties meaning that they find it increasingly hard to cope with the range of people, events, messages, sights and sounds that we are bombarded with all the time. We should recognise the need to avoid over-stimulating the person, for example, by inviting them for a meal with just one or two other people rather than a large party.

> 'Four years on from diagnosis, I have more difficulty decoding what I hear, my balance is shaky and I sometimes forget things like turning off the cooker. I do not enjoy being in large groups, and I cannot stand loud noise.' (Person with dementia)

It is also possible that the person may be experiencing depression – up to a quarter of people with dementia may become depressed at some time during their illness. We should not be afraid to ask the person how they are feeling and help them get support if necessary. People with dementia who become depressed can be offered psychological treatments to help them talk about their feelings and manage symptoms.

## Acceptance

This is our final key principle for family members and friends of a person with early dementia. We need to learn to accept the person's changing abilities, manner and behaviour if the person is to remain socially included. We have already mentioned qualities such as patience, tact and having an unprovoking manner when interacting with the person on a day-to-day basis. We must accept that repetition, forgetfulness, self-absorption and other challenges are all part of the person's growing difficulties, and we must learn to adapt to them and live with them.

'Honesty, patience and an understanding amongst my family and friends is a great help. I don't deal well with confrontation and questioning.' (Person with dementia)

'Give people time; let them do things in their own way and don't take over if it hasn't been done "properly". You need to learn to ask yourself, "Does it really matter?"' (Family member)

### How to offer support

It is important that we learn to accept that the person is changing and that we need to adapt our view of the person accordingly. This can be hard for some family members and friends to do. For example, Mike was a successful businessman, but now has dementia. He attends a day centre regularly, but believes that when the transport comes to take him there, he is going to a business meeting and insists on taking his briefcase and a notebook with him. This upsets Mike's wife Mary, who tries to stop him from doing so – 'You don't need that where you're going', she says. This, in turn, upsets Mike. Surely it would be better for Mary to accept that this is how Mike understands and copes with his situation and let him take his briefcase if he wants to.

> 'I think my mum feels a huge responsibility for grandma, being an only child. She drives herself crazy worrying about what grandma's eating and I know her diet's not ideal but she's happy... I don't think it's worth having the argument with her over something you can't change. It's about being as patient as you can and picking your fights as the saying goes. My mum has a tendency to pick up on everything with my grandma and I just don't see the point of that as it puts her in a bad mood and stresses you out.' (Family member)

Accepting that the person is changing can also help us to resist the urge to avoid the person because 'it isn't really her'. In some ways that might be true, in that their behaviour and outlook may have changed, but ultimately it is the person – the mother, father, aunt, uncle, husband, wife or friend – we have always known and loved.

Another aspect of acceptance is that family members and friends may need to help the person be accepted by others who may not have the same level of understanding or tolerance of people with dementia. We have talked about the stigma that society may display towards people with dementia and the negative stereotype of dementia that can sometimes be expressed in the media. There may be people within the person's family or circle of friends who find it hard to accept that the person should continue to be part of social occasions or activities. We can help through providing a good example of acceptance, or sometimes by tactfully offering information about dementia to those whose understanding may not be as complete as ours.

> 'Sometimes in the evening they'd wander to the local pub and they'd have a drink, just one, and then wander back, and people in the local community always said, "Oh your dad was marvellous with your mum", and they would make a fuss of

my mum and that was good for dad, it got him out of the house and my mum would respond. Even when she didn't have any conversation she would smile at people – for him it was trying to keep a bit of normality in the changing situation.' (Family member)

## PLANNING FOR THE FUTURE

'If I'd known more about what to expect, my husband and I could have had a whale of a time whilst it was possible. We would have been able to plan ahead.' (Family member)

Once dementia has been diagnosed, it is important that the person, their family and friends make plans for the future. This is called *advance care planning*, a process used to help people with dementia plan and record future wishes and priorities of care with those close to them. Dementia will inevitably progress, and key decisions will have to be made regarding such matters as how the person's financial affairs will be managed, where the person will live as their ability to be independent declines and what kind of medical treatment and care the person should receive as they approach the end of life. As dementia progresses, the person will lose the capacity to make those decisions for themselves. If that is the case and the person has not expressed their views in advance, then family members and/or professionals will have to decide for the person, in the person's best interests. The decision-making process can, however, be made much easier if discussions have taken place before the person loses capacity, so that the person can express their views as to how they would like the rest of their life to proceed.

'Don't wait for the future to happen because when it happens you're upset, you're distraught, you don't want to be making the big decisions then.' (Family member)

> 'Me and my daughters have discussed what I want in the future. It turned out they were both polar opposites in what they thought I wanted. Imagine the distress I would have caused that I couldn't put right if we hadn't talked!' (Person with dementia)

Such discussions with family members and friends may be informal and unstructured. Family members often say to professionals, 'We talked about it and this is what he would have wanted.' Professionals should take note of such remembered conversations when making decisions, but it is better if the person sets out their views formally in a structured way. In the UK there are two legal mechanisms for a person with dementia to have their wishes taken into account: *advance decision to refuse treatment (ADRT)* and *power of attorney*. *Advance statements*, whilst not legally binding, are another way for people to express their views and are equally important as they can help provide valuable information about how people would like to be cared for.

> 'I want to know more about the future because I want to enable it to work for me and my wife. But on the other hand, I think, "Sod it", the future's the future, let's live in the day. To be honest, I think both.' (Person with dementia)

## Advance decision to refuse treatment (ADRT)

An ADRT (sometimes known as an advance directive) is a legally drawn-up statement of the person's wish to refuse certain future medical treatments should they lack capacity to make decisions at the time they need those treatments. The person may decide that they do not want to have treatments such as specific drugs or surgery that would prolong their life, feeding tubes, or cardio-pulmonary resuscitation if they have a cardiac arrest. So long as they are valid and applicable, advance decisions are generally legally binding on professionals. A person can only draw up an advance decision for themselves and must have mental capacity when doing so, which will include many people with early dementia.

Advance decisions must be drawn up with care so that doctors and nurses in the future have clear guidelines to follow. An advance decision might say: 'I do not want any form of surgery if I am near the end of my life.' However, it is possible that the person may be in extreme pain and surgery could make their last months easier for them. It is recommended that people compiling an advance decision look carefully at how it is worded, and seek medical and legal advice.

## Advance statements

This is a more general statement of wishes and preferences for treatment or care should the person lose capacity. For example, someone may express a preference for being looked after at home – or state that they would prefer to enter residential care. An advance statement may include information that will help others in looking after that person, such as how they want to be cared for and preferences for activities. They may set out the person's wishes for particular religious rites at the end of life. Unlike advance directives, advance statements are not legally binding, but professionals must take them into account when planning care and treatment.

## Power of attorney

This principle states that a person can legally appoint another to look after their financial affairs, and/or make other decisions on their behalf once they lack capacity to do so. These decisions may embrace consent to medical treatment, deciding where the person should live and so on. It is legally possible for someone with early dementia (so long as they still have mental capacity) to nominate a family member or friend to take on power of attorney. In England and Wales (the process is different in Scotland and Northern Ireland), the legal framework is known as a *lasting power of attorney (LPA)* and comes in two forms:

- Property and financial affairs

- Health and welfare.

Taking out a power of attorney related to financial and property matters has obvious advantages in that the attorney can use the person's money to manage their financial affairs and help pay for support and care when the person themselves is unable to do so. It can also help people with dementia living alone avoid being exploited by unscrupulous tradespeople who may try to sell them things or services that they do not need, and which would become a financial burden to them. Should the person enter residential care, their attorney will be able to manage and dispose of their property, if necessary.

Many people just take out an LPA related to finance and property, but the person can also nominate an attorney to make decisions on their behalf regarding their health and welfare if they lack capacity. Professionals must legally gain permission from the attorney for medical treatments and care decisions regarding the person.

The legal processes needed to set up an advance decision or LPA are involved and complex, and so they should be – the potential for an LPA to be abused or an advance decision to be misinterpreted is considerable. Whilst it is possible so draw up an advance decision or apply for an LPA oneself, many people opt to consult a solicitor to assist with the legal process, and some law firms specialise in such work.

The consequences of not setting up an LPA whilst the person still has capacity can be problematic for family and friends. If the person loses capacity without an LPA in place, no one can legally manage their financial affairs or make health-related decisions on their behalf. A family member or friend would have to apply to the Court of Protection to become a *deputy*. In this role they would have the same legal powers as an attorney under an LPA, but it is a longer and more complex process, and deputies are scrutinised by the Court of Protection in ways that attorneys are not. It is better to avoid the stress (and expense) of applying for a deputyship by encouraging the person to set up an LPA whilst they still have capacity. The benefits of doing so also include clarifying the person's wishes whilst they are still able to express them, and avoiding potential misunderstanding or disagreement between family members.

Although conversations about future wishes can be difficult to consider early on in the diagnosis, they are extremely important. It is also important to review advance care planning documents on a regular basis, as preferences and wishes can change. Further guidance and examples of advance care planning documents can be found in the Resources section at the end of the book.

> 'My LPA is filed away and every now and then my daughters will ask me to confirm it's still what I want, and then it's filed away again.' (Person with dementia)

## COMPILING A LIFE STORY

A life story is a very practical way that family members and friends may support a person with early dementia and assist them to prepare for the future. It is exactly what it sounds like: a history or story of the person's life to date. The resulting life story could take many forms; many are in the form of books filled with photographs, written accounts, letters, certificates and so on that together tell the story of the person's life. Some people use digital media when putting together a life story, compiling photograph shows or videos. Life story albums are also being developed on social media internet sites such as Facebook and YouTube.

There is a clear advantage in compiling a life story during the early years, when the person can contribute to deciding what goes into the story and can appreciate the result. However, life stories can be compiled by family members, friends or professional carers at any time, but must be as inclusive as possible, and be based on a good understanding of the person's preferences and wishes. Life stories are valuable in a number of ways:

- They can help people with dementia reflect on their lives, share their story and enhance their sense of identity. This is especially useful when people have difficulty in sharing this information themselves.

- They can help the person develop closer relationships with family members and others through sharing their story.

- If, in the future, the person attends a day centre or care home, staff will find a life story invaluable for becoming better acquainted with the person as a person, and will be able to see them as an individual with a rich past.

- It may also help them understand the person's manner and behaviour better if they can relate that behaviour to aspects of the person's past life (see Chapter 8).

There are various short templates used in hospitals and care homes that can provide a snapshot of the things that are most important to that person. These should not replace life story work, but can be a useful accessible resource for staff in getting to know someone and ensuring their needs are met. See the Resources section for some examples.

As stated above, if compiled in the early years of dementia when the person still has some awareness, the person can contribute and decide themselves what goes into their life story and what is left out. There may be particular aspects of their life that the person would prefer to be left unrecorded, such as events that were upsetting or that have been kept secret. It does not matter if a life story is not complete; it is more important that it reflects and celebrates the person's life. Written biographies are always selective, presenting the person in a particular way, and there is no reason why a life story should be any different.

> 'I need to do a "This is me" document some time soon to take into hospital if need be.' (Family member)

## INTIMACY AND SEXUALITY

Many people with early dementia live with their spouse or partner and will have been used to intimate and sexual relationships. Frequently, sexual relationships continue into old age. The question then arises: what should happen to intimacy and sexual relationships if one partner develops dementia?

If the person retains awareness and mental capacity, there should not be an issue, as the person has the ability to consent to sexual relationships and those relationships can continue as before. But what if the person's awareness of their condition seems to be declining and their capacity to make decisions is compromised? Let us consider an example of a married couple who have always enjoyed sex. The wife develops dementia but retains awareness in the early phase and still participates willingly in sexual activities. But then dementia progresses and she lacks the capacity to make decisions in most situations. However, she still responds positively when her husband makes sexual overtures towards her, and they continue to have sex and she seems to enjoy it. Is this right, or might her husband be sexually exploiting or even abusing her?

We would argue that this does not have to be the case. If a person cannot give consent for an activity in the strict sense of the word, they can still display willingness to participate in that activity, and we can gauge that willingness by their actions, words and mood – if they actually take part in the activity, say they are enjoying it and appear content and happy, then we may assume they are willing to do it. As we will see in subsequent chapters, the principle of willingness provides the basis for carrying out a whole range of social and recreational activities with people with more advanced dementia, and we believe it can equally apply to a husband and wife's sexual activities – we can assume that the wife is willing because of her actions, words and mood, and because they match how she has always responded to her husband's sexual advances. However, care must always be taken as dementia progresses to ensure that the person is indeed still willing, because if there is any indication of coercion or distress as a result of sexual activity, this would be considered a criminal act.

The situation becomes more complex if, as sometimes happens, the onset of dementia leads to a change in the person's level of interest in sexual activities. If they become less interested, then their partner should respect that – empathy means that we need to appreciate that the change derives from the person's dementia and we should accept and adapt to that change. If the person's level of interest increases, problems can arise if their partner does not wish to have more sex, and within the relationship the situation will have to be resolved the best way it can – whether or not a person in a relationship has dementia, sex should only take place within that relationship if both partners are willing for it to happen.

> 'Previously we both instigated intimacy, but dementia changed that. He once accused me of raping him, so I will not put myself into that situation again.' (Family member)

More challenging still is the case where dementia leads to the person making sexual overtures towards others. If the person is unattached and the individual they make advances to is attracted to the person, is it right for them to respond? Would the principle of willingness apply in this case? We are not so sure – the potential for exploitation and abuse is perhaps too great. Also, suppose for a moment that the person is suddenly cured of their dementia and realises how they had been acting. The chances are that the person would be embarrassed, ashamed or horrified. In some cases it is more appropriate for us to adopt a 'paternalistic' approach towards people with dementia when their behaviour may cause distress to others, or would cause themselves distress if they became aware of what they were doing.

> 'I would really like to talk to someone about sexual relations. It's a big hole in the literature and seems to get glossed over. I don't know how to approach it, as it was an important part

of our relationship. I try to find ways of staying intimate but sometimes this doesn't work, which feels like another loss.' (Family member)

## ASSISTIVE TECHNOLOGY

We have considered above ways that the person may be assisted to compensate for increasing memory loss and difficulties in completing complex tasks through the use of lists, reminders and labels and clearly set out instructions. All these strategies will, of course, enhance the person's ability to remain independent. In the early phase, when the person retains awareness, they may well be able to devise their own memory-supporting strategies. To complement such approaches, the concept of assistive technology has been developed. This is the use of both low- and high-tech devices to help people remain independent and reduce the risks of them coming to harm. Assistive technology is not new – anyone who wears spectacles or has a hearing aid or a walking stick is using assistive technology.

'Using a stick, to help with balance and perception problems, distance and height such as curbs and steps. My stick is also a visual aid to others that I might need assistance or support when my problems aren't always seen.' (Person with dementia)

Slightly more sophisticated are items such as calendar clocks that display the date as well as the time, which some people with dementia find useful for keeping track of days of the week. We have previously mentioned mobile phones as useful aids for the person to keep in touch with family and friends, offering the opportunity of giving the person quick reminders through text messaging or allowing the person to phone someone if they get into difficulties when out of the house.

Some more specialised technological aids are available for people with early dementia. Examples include computerised reminders, such as a device that gives the person a message when they are about to leave the house to remind them to take their door key. Safety technology includes heat or flood detectors, or devices that automatically switch off gas taps if the person leaves them on. Leisure devices include easy-to-use radios and music players. Another aspect of assistive technology is the use of tracking devices that are worn by the person and use GPS technology, so that the person's whereabouts can be known at all times. Such technology may allow a person with dementia to go out on their own and be recovered if they get lost.

'My daughters used to worry about me travelling, but because we talk, we were able to find a solution. So now they track me and it makes them feel safer and me feel happier.' (Person with dementia)

Yet another new development is the increased interest of some health and social care authorities in establishing support based on electronic devices that are placed around the person's house to monitor anything that may compromise the person's safety, such as gas leaks, floods and fire, or if the person has fallen or gone out of the house unexpectedly. These devices are connected to a central monitoring point and alarms are raised if the system reports anything untoward.

Assistive technology has clear benefits if it is successful in assisting a person to live independently and safely, and its use can offer considerable reassurance to family and friends. However, it is not a panacea, and a number of drawbacks have been identified:

- It can work for some people but not others; for example, one person may understand and respond to computerised reminders whilst another may be more confused by them. All technology is complex, and dementia may quickly compromise a person's ability to relate to it.

- Assistive technology devices can be expensive and may not be available for free from the state.

- There has been some debate about the use of tracking aids due to concern that they may compromise privacy and human rights. However, such debate also considered that they can help support risk enablement, and discussions with people with dementia indicate this is in their best interests and not an infringement of rights. Most importantly, any decision about using such devices should be taken based on knowing the person, thinking about their capacity, and balancing risks with independence. It is possible that the person could give permission for such devices to be used as part of an advance decision.

Assistive technologies can bring great reassurance to family and friends that someone is safe, especially when they are not nearby. However, they should not be seen as a replacement for social contact. A number of useful information sources can be found in the Resources section.

## DRIVING

This is an aspect of daily life that can create great anxiety for family members and friends. There is no intrinsic reason why a person with early dementia cannot continue to drive if they retain awareness and ability – a diagnosis of dementia does not automatically exclude a person from having a driving licence in the UK, although the diagnosis would have to be declared to the DVLA and insurers. Once notified, people are usually required to undertake a test to ensure they are still safe to drive, and some specialist testing centres are available. However, the progression of dementia will inevitably compromise the person's ability to drive safely. Growing memory loss can lead to difficulty with remembering routes or the meaning of road signs. Attention deficits will affect ability to concentrate on the road and notice potential hazards, and executive function impairment will compromise the person's ability to make appropriate decisions whilst driving. Sometimes a person with dementia can continue to drive for a while if someone is with them to give directions and point out hazards, but sooner or later the point is reached when it is realised that the person could harm themselves or others if they continue to attempt to drive.

'I only drive short distances and not at night, and I am happy to be the passenger when my wife is in the car.' (Person with dementia)

'My husband would drive along in low gears or wouldn't change down gears and didn't understand why the car was juddering. We'd have to tell him to change gear.' (Family member)

Giving up driving can be traumatic for the person and for their family and friends. Sometimes the person realises themselves that they can't cope at the wheel and gives up driving voluntarily, or acquiesces to family members' entreaties that they should not drive.

'My husband drove to a nearby town which is only a seven-mile journey that he had done for 30 years, and couldn't find his way home. He came home having driven around for three hours, unable to find a single landmark that he recognised. He came in in a cold sweat, and threw the keys on the table saying, "Never let me drive again!"' (Family member)

But in some cases, driving is brought to an end by the person having an accident or being stopped by the police and their licence taken away following a driving assessment. When some people with dementia lack awareness that their driving abilities are no longer acceptable and refuse to give up driving, how should families respond in such cases?

Some family members in these circumstances resort to acts of deception to prevent the person driving. They may hide the car keys and pretend to the person they have been lost. They may remove the battery leads so that the car cannot start, or they may even sell the car, telling the person it had been written off in an accident. Is it right to use deceptions such as these with people with dementia? Some would say that deception in any circumstance is ethically wrong; it dehumanises the person, and if they find out they have been lied to, it can make the situation worse. On the other hand, others would feel that deception in this situation is worth it to prevent the person harming themselves or others by continuing to drive. They would point out that deception is a fact of life – how often do we tell half-truths or white lies or keep things to ourselves as part of our everyday relationships with others? We will consider the role of truth telling and deception in dementia care further in Chapter 6.

## WHERE SHOULD A PERSON WITH EARLY DEMENTIA LIVE?

Many people with dementia who live in 'the community' live with their spouse, who is most likely to take on the main caring role for the person. With dementia affecting in the main people at the older end of the age spectrum, the person's spouse is likely to be themselves elderly. Others live with their adult children – who may well be in their 50s and 60s or older – and a significant number live alone. This is likely to reflect their own preference, and they may well manage effectively in their own familiar surroundings, with the support of family and friends. We have discussed above the strategies and aids for helping a person with dementia maintain independence, and whilst these do not exclusively apply to people with dementia who live alone, they clearly have considerable potential value to those people. But what if dementia has progressed to the point where despite such supports the person may be at risk of harm from neglect, accident or possible exploitation?

Part of the answer may be enhanced professional support that can help the person remain in their own home (see Chapter 4). But sooner or later a specific question may arise for a relative or close friend of a person with dementia: should my relative or friend come to live with me?

It may seem obvious that a person with early dementia who finds it difficult to live alone but who does not need or want residential care should go to live with a close relative or friend, especially when it is a son or daughter, and this is what many people do. However, it is not a decision to be taken lightly, and families considering such a move have many factors to weigh up in coming to that decision. First, is it what the person with dementia wants? Many would find such a move comforting and would enjoy the company, but some would prefer not to burden others or would find life in a younger family noisy and difficult. Second, is the family prepared for the extra responsibility and potential stress of having a person with dementia in the household, even if it is a loved parent? Research shows that adult children caring for a person with dementia in their household experience more stress than other carers. It can change their lives: adult children may find themselves having to give up work in order to look after their parent – caring for a person with dementia can have greater financial implications than other forms of caring. Previously difficult family relationships may resurface, leading to conflict, and if the adult child has their own children still at home, they might be torn between their needs and the needs of their parent.

Alternatively there can be many positives for families and friends in taking people into their own homes, such as maintaining relationships, giving something back and gaining satisfaction from the caring role. The stresses are very real, though, and it is important that decisions to make such arrangements are thought through very carefully. Possible alternatives such as supported accommodation or paid care at home should also be considered with the person before making a decision.

## THE CASE FOR IMPROVING SUPPORT SERVICES DURING THE EARLY YEARS OF DEMENTIA

Research is increasingly suggesting that minimising support services during the years of early dementia due to financial constraints may be a false economy. People with dementia and their families who receive particular forms of support or input may do better than those who do not, with the person maybe progressing through dementia at a slower rate, and families being able to manage caring for the person for longer. Specific interventions that have been shown by research to have such benefits but that are not always available include the following:

- *Psycho-social interventions* carried out by some community practitioners, such as psychologists or Admiral Nurses, including specific education, counselling and stress management interventions, can improve family members' ability to care for the person with dementia and enhance their emotional coping resources. They may also reduce rates of admission to residential care.

- *Cognitive stimulation techniques* for people with early dementia, sometimes carried out individually with the person and sometimes within group sessions, may, according to some research, be as good as or better than AChE inhibitor drugs in slowing the progression of dementia, and may improve the person's mood.

- *Care management* in which there is a named person that the person with dementia and their family can contact, and who oversees and coordinates their care, is recommended as it can help ensure people get the right information and access to support, improve continuity for families and prevent crises happening.

Families and friends sometimes feel that they have been left to their own devices, and that more information and support in the early months or years of dementia may have eased the journey as dementia progressed. We may help by supporting campaigns that are seeking to improve the provision of professional support available for those with early dementia.

> 'You need to have someone who can coordinate things for you and who understands the system...someone to talk to – a point of contact who knows about what you are going through and understands your situation.' (Family member)

# CHAPTER 6

# Managing Change as Dementia Progresses

## HOW DEMENTIA PROGRESSES

The rate that dementia progresses will vary markedly from person to person. Some people may, with the right support, maintain relative independence for quite a few years. For others the progression of the condition appears more marked, and a noticeable decline in function may be observed after a relatively short period of time. Sooner or later, however, people with dementia come to experience some characteristic difficulties. These may be present regardless of the actual type of dementia, as by this time most common forms of dementia are beginning to share similarities:

- Memory problems will usually be more profound, with increased difficulty in remembering new information. Memories for past life may begin to be impaired. Some things may be forgotten completely, whilst other things may become muddled or half remembered. This can lead to the person believing things that are not now the case, such as that they are still going to work or that a long-dead relative is still alive.

- The person may have lost awareness of their condition and have limited understanding that there is anything amiss.

- The person may have problems with understanding complex concepts. Reading books and hobbies or activities that involve complex reasoning, such as some card games, quizzes or crosswords, may be too difficult.

- The person's orientation to their surroundings can become more impaired. They may have problems with finding their way around safely in unfamiliar surroundings or with understanding the time or date and not know what season of the year it is. They will usually still recognise significant people such as family members and friends, but may not remember or recognise less familiar others.

- For some people, language abilities may become more impaired. If this happens, sentence construction can be compromised and the person may have increased difficulty with word finding. Whilst they should still be able to understand what others say to them, so long as the message isn't too complex, they may well have difficulty responding. Often the content of what they say may be limited to simple ideas and be repetitive.

- The person's ability to attend to events or concentrate for long periods can be compromised. Their interest in other people may appear to reduce, although this is more to do with memory, comprehension and attention difficulties than unsociability.

- Changes in emotion or manner may become apparent and tend to be expressed through the way the person behaves. Some people become very passive and withdrawn, whilst others appear restless and agitated at times, and may be prone to outbursts of agitation or frustration. Some people appear to have a great need for physical activity and walking about. People may also say things or behave in a way that appears hurtful or insensitive. This can be particularly difficult for close family or friends, and is addressed in more detail in Chapter 8.

- The person is likely to begin to find daily living activities more difficult. They may have problems preparing meals or drinks for themselves. Most people will still be able to eat and drink without assistance, although preferences for food may change – for example, they may come to prefer sweeter or spicy food. They are likely still to be able to wash and dress themselves, but may get muddled, putting clothes on in the wrong order or forgetting particular things. They may begin to have difficulties with using the toilet, leading to occasional accidents.

- Unless they have unrelated physical health problems, the person is still likely to be physically well and active, and can usually get about without assistance other than finding their way in unfamiliar places. However, for some people who have visual-perceptual difficulties, there may be problems with recognising and interpreting their environment. For example, patterns on floors, poor lighting, mirrors and ill-defined contrasts between walls and doors may cause the person difficulties with moving about.

These problems are related to how the person understands the world around them and/or is able to respond. Appreciating the specific difficulties that the person has and trying to see the world the way the person sees it will help us interact with and support the person more effectively.

By now, many people will struggle to live on their own, unless they have regular support from family members, friends or professionals. More likely they will be living with a 'main carer', often a spouse, partner or adult child. Some may be able to live in sheltered or supported accommodation with professional support. Some families may, by this time, be considering residential care for the person or that transition may have been made. We consider the specific issues around residential care in Chapter 9.

## THE CHANGING NATURE OF RELATIONSHIPS

Family members and friends will become acutely aware of the fact that their relationship with the person is changing, with that relationship becoming increasingly less equal as the person's condition progresses. Family members in particular can experience a sense of loss, known as *anticipatory grief.*

'My disease has certainly upset my wife. She (like me) feels bereaved of what she had looked forward to or expected.' (Person with dementia)

'It feels like my husband's disappearing – for example, he says things that are not in character. It's losing someone: I feel like I'm being widowed before he's gone. It's like living with someone that you don't know, but at other times I get a reminder of our closeness.' (Family member)

The person may find it harder to respond to others as they used to. They may appear less interested in other people's lives or concerns and be less able to show or reciprocate affection. Social situations can become difficult to cope with and they may become distressed or want to avoid them. If the person has noticeably changed, it can be harder for family members and friends to recognise the person as they once were, particularly regarding their cognitive abilities and sometimes their manner as well. These changes are likely to be distressing for family and friends. The temptation to avoid the person may become great for those not obliged to directly care for the person, and friends may become increasingly distant, especially if behaviour changes.

Those who have adopted the role of 'main carer' will feel most profoundly the change in the nature of their relationship with the person. A spouse or long-term partner who was used to an equal relationship of mutual interdependence will have to come to terms with the person with dementia depending on them more. An adult child who may have relied, to an extent, on their parent for support and help throughout their life may now have to provide that support and help themselves. There is no easy way for family members and friends to come to terms with the relationship changes that come with the progression of dementia. Above all, it is important to accept that the person has changed, and whilst we can still recognise aspects of them as the person they were and hold onto this, we also need to accept the differences that dementia can bring.

'As I need more support from my daughters, relinquishing my independence is one of my greatest fears. I don't want dementia to impact greatly on their lives.' (Person with dementia)

Mutual support remains crucial, as does trying to maintain an attitude of wanting the best for the person, and helping them to lead as satisfying a life as possible. For family members or friends who are providing direct care, it is essential to accept support from others, both practically and emotionally, especially as the needs of the person with dementia become greater. The temptation may be to 'soldier on' and to try to cope as it can be difficult to ask for help, but it is really important to look after your own needs and to share the caring.

'Other friends have become closer and offer to sit with my husband, and that's really important.' (Family member)

The person's growing difficulties also mean that family members and friends must learn to interact with them in a new way. This is represented in the figure below.

Normal relationships can be expressed in this simple form:

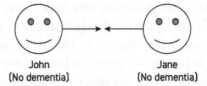

John
(No dementia)

Jane
(No dementia)

When both people have similar abilities, their communication is equal and reciprocal – both can reach out to each other and expect a response. But now consider a relationship between John and Mary, who has difficulties as a result of her dementia progressing:

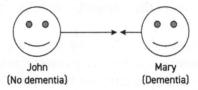

John
(No dementia)

Mary
(Dementia)

People whose dementia has progressed cannot reach out to others in the same way. This means that John must make more effort to reach out and have a relationship with Mary. This may be reflected in the way that John interacts with Mary. The psychologist Tom Kitwood expressed it thus: 'The quality of interaction is warmer, richer in feeling, than that of everyday life.'

A word of caution is needed, however, when communicating with people who need more help. Communicating in a way that reaches out to them does not mean speaking to someone as though they are unable to understand or as you might speak to a child. There is a clear risk of being patronising or condescending, which is likely to upset someone rather than make them feel acknowledged, included and respected. This is addressed in more detail below.

'I'd want to feel the emotion and be part of it. I don't want to be patted on the head and spoken to in a condescending manner. Wherever possible I want people to treat me the way they treat me now.' (Person with dementia)

## COMMUNICATION AND LANGUAGE AS DEMENTIA PROGRESSES

Human relationships are expressed through communication and language, and it is with impairments in the person's ability to communicate effectively that the progression of dementia is most evident. Learning to understand what a person with dementia is trying to communicate, and knowing how best to respond to the person, is a key task for family members and friends.

> 'No one knows what it's like to be trapped inside there, not being able to express oneself any longer.' (Person with dementia)

Language is, of course, central to communication, but communication is more than language. Much of our communication with others is done para-verbally, through the way we speak, or non-verbally, through our manner and actions. This is even more the case with a person whose dementia has progressed, whose verbal language abilities may be compromised. As we will see in Chapter 8, much of the behaviour of people with dementia that others find difficult is likely to represent the person's attempt to communicate non-verbally needs and wishes that they cannot express through language.

### Language difficulties as dementia progresses

As described in Chapter 3, there are some specific types of dementia, known as *semantic dementia*, that tend to affect speech more than other functions. However, for other, more common types of dementia, the person's language and communication difficulties will largely reflect the more global difficulties of dementia. As memory deficits and decline of cognitive abilities become more profound, the person may say less or their conversation may include muddled memories or become very repetitive. Also, the person may not understand abstract ideas, and can mistake those talking to them with someone else, perhaps a significant family member from the past. Growing attention issues make it harder for the person to concentrate on what others are saying to them, and impairment of executive function may mean that the person struggles to follow simple instructions. Sometimes the person may seem to be talking to someone, which can be due to visual hallucinations – seeing people or things that are not there. The person may also display difficulties with communication that reflect damage to the language areas of the brain, such as word-finding problems. For those who have 'semantic dementia', which affects the temporal lobes of the brain, specific problems include remembering the meaning of words, faces and objects. The person may know what they want to say but cannot put their message into a coherent form – we tend to label what they are saying as 'rambling' or 'confused' talk, but it clearly means something to the person. Sometimes they display *perseveration*, a tendency to repeat the same word or phrase over and over, like a stuck record. Understanding what may be behind the person's language difficulties is the first step to becoming able to communicate with them effectively.

## How *not* to communicate with a person with dementia

As indicated earlier, there are many mistakes we can make when communicating with people whose dementia has progressed. These mistakes matter, because if the person perceives them, they can increase the person's sense of ill-being or lack of worth. The psychologist Tom Kitwood researched into this area and identified common communication errors that he termed *malignant social psychology*. His research was carried out with professional care staff, but family members and friends may well recognise some of their own ways of interacting with the person in Kitwood's categories – although it should be noted that the following is not a complete list:

- *Infantilisation:* Addressing a person very patronisingly, as an insensitive person might treat a young child.

- *Outpacing:* Providing information, presenting choices, etc. at a rate too fast for the person to understand; putting them under pressure to do things more rapidly than they can bear.

- *Ignoring:* Carrying on a conversation in the presence of a person, as if they were not there.

- *Accusation:* Blaming a person for actions or failures of action that arise from their lack of ability or their misunderstanding of the situation.

- *Mockery:* Making fun of the person's 'strange' actions or remarks; teasing, humiliating, making jokes at their expense.

- *Disparagement:* Telling a person they are incompetent, useless or worthless, or otherwise giving them messages that are damaging to their self-esteem.

How many of these communication errors did you recognise and, if you are honest, have found yourself making – or heard others make? We have observed that people with dementia may well retain the ability to understand what is said to them, long after their ability to communicate verbally themselves has been lost, and if the person heard and understood a family member or friend communicating in these ways it would clearly upset them, even if they could not always express that upset.

A famous quote by Maya Angelou helps illustrate the importance of attending to how we communicate: 'I've learned that people will forget what you said, people will forget what you did, but people will never forget how you made them feel.'

## LISTENING AND RESPONDING TO A PERSON WITH COMMUNICATION DIFFICULTIES

People with dementia want to talk and interact, and family members and friends should encourage them to do so. To the extent that their communications are understandable and reflect reality, we can respond to them just as we would if they did not have dementia. As the condition progresses, however, the person's speech may display some of the impairments described earlier. How should we respond to the person in these cases? We will consider two of the most common situations that may arise: when the person expresses unreal beliefs or different realities and when the person's speech is muddled.

### Responding when the person expresses unreal beliefs or different realities

A recent report by the Mental Health Foundation, called the *Truth Inquiry*, explored the issue of unreal beliefs or different realities experienced by people with dementia and offered some useful guidance on how best to both understand and respond to these. Further information can be found in the Resources section at the end of the book. Here we use the principles offered in the *Truth Inquiry* to help us think about how best to communicate when people are experiencing what is described as a *different reality*. Examples of how someone with dementia might display different realities include:

- Believing that a significant person from the past, such as a parent, is still alive

- Being convinced that a family member or friend is someone different, or is deceiving them

- Not recognising their own home and asking to 'go home', believing home is elsewhere

- Believing they are still in a previous role and wanting to carry out related activities

- Wanting to do something not in keeping with their previous religion or beliefs

- Feeling scared or persecuted by things or people that are not there, or feeling that people are 'out to get them'.

It is important to understand why the person might be feeling or behaving in this way.

First, as stated above, if memory impairment is profound, the person may well find that their remaining memories are muddled, or they may mix up their memories of the past with the present. This can lead to them believing things to be true that are no longer the case. This is sometimes referred to as *time-shifting*, as longer-term memories are often easier to recall than more recent ones. This may be useful for the person in trying to make sense of the world around them and providing a sense of security.

Second, some different realities can be a way of someone expressing a feeling or unmet need, such as feeling bored, frustrated, lost or scared. Alternatively, the person may be experiencing problems with interpreting their environment due to perceptual difficulties or hallucinations and delusions as a feature of their dementia. (It is also important to note that hallucinations and delusions are a common symptom of delirium, and if there is a sudden change in the person's behaviour, this should be considered as a possible cause – see Chapter 3.) These experiences are often distressing for people, and great sensitivity is required in responding.

Last, we should also consider that what the person is saying may actually be true. For example, if someone is accusing people of stealing from them and they have people coming into their home, we should not automatically assume that this is not the case and they are misinterpreting things due to their dementia. Whatever the cause, it is important to remember that this communication will have some meaning for the person and should not be dismissed.

So how should we respond when someone is experiencing a different reality? For example, when a person with dementia says:

- 'Is my mother coming to see me today?' (when the person's mother has died)

- 'I need to leave now as I need to get to work' (when the person has retired)

- 'Why are you in my house? Where is my wife?' (when the person is no longer recognising their family member).

Do we tell them the absolute truth and remind them of reality? Do we 'go along' with their reality? Do we use what is sometimes referred to as a 'white lie' in response?

There is no easy answer to this question. We could argue that in everyday life people are not always completely truthful with each other. For example, how do we respond when a close friend or family member asks us: 'Does my bum look big in this?' We may not always respond completely truthfully if we know that an honest response might cause them upset!

Whilst in dementia some communication may have less basis in reality, the same principles of knowing the person and understanding what is important to them should influence our response. Useful questions to consider include:

- How meaningful is this different reality for the person?

- Are they trying to express something to us, for example feeling scared, frustrated or lost?

- How much distress is it causing?

Such situations can also be very distressing for family members or friends, and our own feelings can influence how we respond.

Ultimately, responses should be informed by doing everything we can to understand what is behind the communication and how best to support the well-being of the person. The *Truth Inquiry* recommends some key principles to underpin responses to the expression of different realities:

- Different realities are often meaningful for the person.

- We should do everything we can to find out the meaning.

- Responses should be underpinned by kindness, compassion, respect and understanding.

- Start with the principle of truth telling – but use an alternative approach or 'untruth' if you know the truth is likely to cause distress.

- Lies should only be used if alternative responses are not helpful and are needed to avoid acute distress.

- Responses should be consistent between carers, family and friends if possible.

The range of possible responses may be regarded as falling on a continuum from truth to lies. We offer the following, adapted from the *Truth Inquiry*, to help consider different ways of responding if a person says, 'Is my mother coming to see me today?'

| Whole truth telling | Alternative responses | | Untruths | | Lying |
|---|---|---|---|---|---|
| | Looking for alternative meanings | Reframing/ validating | Distracting | 'Going along with' | |
| 'I'm sorry, your mother died a long time ago' | 'Is everything okay? Is there a particular reason you need to see your mother?' | 'It sounds like you miss your mother. Can you tell me more about her?' | 'Sorry, she's not here. Why don't we have a cup of tea?' | 'I'm sorry but she can't come to see you today' | 'Don't worry, she'll be here soon' |

### Whole truth telling
As illustrated above, we could correct the person and tell them, 'Sorry, your mother won't be coming as she died 10 years ago.' Some would label this kind of response as *reality orientation*

and would say that it is appropriate that people with dementia are assisted to keep in touch with current reality as much as possible. This may be the case for those people whose memory and awareness is not too impaired, but consider the effect on the person of being given this news – it will at the very least upset them to learn that their mother is dead. It will remind them that they are themselves cognitively impaired as they realise that they have forgotten such a significant event. And if the news is given in a harsh or critical way, the person will feel demeaned and belittled.

Consider also that the person may quickly forget what has been said to them and later on may again ask if their mother is coming to visit. If those around them correct them again, they will experience anew the upset and ill-being that will result. Some have compared this situation to experiencing bereavement over and over.

### Lying

At the other end of the continuum is telling a 'white lie' to the person, such as: 'Don't worry, she'll be here soon.' We have already raised the question of the use of deception with people with dementia. Some people in some situations may regard telling 'white lies' as being acceptable if they help resolve difficult situations such as preventing a person from driving when they are not safe to do so. Is a white lie, in the form of collusion with the person's unreal belief, a helpful response in this case?

One difficulty with this kind of collusion is that once entered into, it is hard for family members and friends to extract themselves from it. They would, in effect, have to maintain the fiction every time the person raises the topic of their mother. Then, if the person becomes impatient or distressed that their mother hasn't yet arrived, another white lie will be needed to try to resolve the situation: 'Oh, she's rung up to say her train's been cancelled and she'll come tomorrow instead.' Alternatively, if someone remembers later that their mother is dead but that others have not told them, it may lead to a breakdown of trust. This may cause the person more distress, and leave family members and friends with bad feelings.

'I have a real problem with the notion of telling "therapeutic lies". Tell me better truths instead.' (Person with dementia)

## Alternative responses

For people who are experiencing different realities, the responses described in the middle of the continuum are probably the most helpful, especially as cognitive abilities decline. We might try one of the 'alternative responses':

- *Looking for alternative meanings:* This involves trying to establish the reason behind what the person is saying. In the example provided, someone asking for their mother may be an indication that they are feeling lost, alone or frightened. They may be feeling unwell or in pain. Mothers often represent a sense of comfort or security, and this need may be what is behind the question.

- *Reframing/validating:* This response involves not agreeing or disagreeing with the person's belief but attempting to engage with the person at the level of the feelings that underlie that belief. As indicated, an example of a validating response in this case would be: 'It sounds like you miss your mum. Can you tell me about her?' Such a response allows the person to talk about their feelings regarding the person from the past whilst hopefully distracting them from the reality that their mother has died. In this way the person's well-being is maintained, and family members and friends can interact with the person in a positive way.

## Untruths

If the above responses do not work, it may be helpful to try one of the approaches below. They do not involve a direct 'lie' but are equally not completely 'true'. Such interactions provide a quick and straightforward means of responding to some potentially awkward situations, and can help make the person feel better.

- *Distracting:* This response can be used to move the person on from the question by offering another activity or topic of conversation. This may be helpful if the person is repeatedly asking the same question and is not prepared to engage in conversation about their feelings. For some people, asking the same question can be a way of asking for contact due to feeling bored or lonely. Offering a cup of tea or an alternative activity can provide them with something to do and contact with someone. However, it is important not to make the person feel you are 'brushing them off' as this may increase their distress rather than make them feel better.

- *'Going along with':* This type of response is often used when someone is more cognitively impaired and a simple solution is required to alleviate distress. It is, of course, not using the truth, but as discussed before, it may be what is needed if other responses don't work. Going along with someone's reality can help to make the person feel valued, offer some comfort and improve their sense of well-being. It may also feel easier for family and friends if they feel they are not 'lying' in the strict sense of the word.

In summary, there are no hard and fast rules about how to respond to unreal beliefs – any of the above approaches may be appropriate in different situations. Having a range of communication skills appropriate for people with dementia will help families and friends maintain close relationships with them.

> 'Treat the person the way you always have and accept their perception of what's going on – it may not be the correct perception but go along with it. Don't contradict – if it isn't going to do harm, why correct it?' (Family member)

## Responding to 'muddled' speech

Another common communication difficulty that people may experience as dementia progresses is when they have something they want to say but cannot express their message properly and their speech appears to others to be 'muddled'.

> 'One time mum tried to tell me something but it had gone and she put her head down and started to cry and I remember taking hold of her hand and saying, "It's okay." She said that what she wanted to say was "there", then she described it as "disappearing". She still had that awareness – she was so upset about it. When she couldn't get the words out right you did a lot of saying "Don't worry mum, it doesn't matter", but it clearly mattered to her.' (Family member)

Bob is being visited by his daughter and baby grandson. He reaches out and takes the baby's hand and says with a smile on his face: 'There now, that'll be a good, er...whatsname isn't it, one day that'll be...whatsit...up here like...won't you be now...' How can we help Bob get his message across?

We could respond by asking Bob to say his message again and he might be able to make it clearer the second time around. However, he may find it even harder to express himself again and may even forget what it was that he wanted to say, leading to possible distress and a breakdown of communication. An alternative strategy that Bob's daughter could employ is to try to find the basic sense within his message, and in a variation of validation, respond to the feelings that Bob is trying to express. Clues to that feeling may come from interpreting what Bob says and also from the way he says it – does he appear happy, sad or angry when making his speech?

In this case we can assume from his smile that Bob is trying to say something happy or jocular. Holding his grandson's hand indicates that the message is about the baby. Clues as to the message can be found in what he has said: '...one day...up here...won't you be...' Bob may be trying to say something like: 'You'll be a big strapping lad one day, won't you!'

If his daughter can pick such clues up, she can make a response that reflects the sense of what Bob is saying: 'He'll be a big boy soon, won't he, Dad!' In this way Bob's feelings are acknowledged, even if the whole of what he wanted to say was not perfectly understood.

## The value of reflection

The case of Bob is an example of the communication technique of *reflection* (sometimes called *mirroring*), which, in this context, means identifying the basic sense of a person's communication and reflecting that sense back to the person. Child care expert Penelope Leach has observed that we use reflection naturally with babies and toddlers – when a youngster says delightedly 'doggy!' we automatically respond, 'Yes, there's a dog, isn't there!', As our children grow older, however, Leach comments that we often give up reflection as a way of interacting, and rarely use it in adulthood. Reflection is, however, a powerful communication technique and forms the basis of many approaches to counselling. Hearing the sense of what we have said gives us a good feeling as we can see that the person has listened enough to be able to repeat the message back to us.

Reflection is a very useful communication technique when interacting with people with dementia. Repeating back their messages gives the person a sense of acknowledgement and validation. Reflection is often best done at a simple level – for example:

Bob: 'Grand – er – thing – day.' [pointing generally outside]

Daughter: 'It's a lovely day outside, isn't it?'

Daughter: 'Are you enjoying your tea, Dad?'

Bob: 'Right tasty. It's ummmm…taste…[smacking his lips]… yes.'

Daughter: 'It tastes nice, does it? That's good.'

Some readers may be wondering why we are advocating a communication technique with people with dementia that we characteristically use with very young children. Isn't this demeaning the person? We were warned above by Tom Kitwood that we should avoid infantilisation as an example of malignant social psychology. We would argue, however, that we are not treating people with dementia in a childlike way if we use techniques such as reflection; we are simply borrowing a communication technique from one setting and applying it to another. This is an example of a transferable skill that many of us will have acquired as parents that may help us interact better with people with dementia.

## GIVING A MESSAGE TO A PERSON WHOSE DEMENTIA HAS PROGRESSED

Family members and friends will often want to give messages to the person they are supporting. They will want to tell them things, ask them things and sometimes give them instructions that will help them carry out tasks and activities. How can we ensure that our messages get through to the person? We will need to use empathy if we are to maximise our chances of the person understanding and responding appropriately to our messages. This means remembering that the person's difficulties will affect attention, memory and executive function, and trying to shape our messages in ways that will compensate for those difficulties.

Let us suppose that Ron, a friend of Bob's, has come to visit him. There are some basic principles that Ron can apply to make his conversation with Bob successful and agreeable to both of them:

- The setting for the conversation should be arranged to assist Bob to attend and concentrate. Lights should be bright but not glaring, and there should be minimal extraneous noises or distractions – remember that people with dementia find it particularly hard to selectively attend if there are too many things happening around them.

- Ron must ensure that Bob has his attention. This means approaching Bob slowly from the front, to give Bob time to focus. If Bob is sitting down and does not appear to have noticed that Ron is there, Ron could crouch down in front of Bob's chair so that Bob can look down at him – research suggests that people with dementia find it easier to attend in those circumstances.

- Ron should not assume that Bob knows who he is, even if Bob appears to recognise him. As we've suggested earlier, people with dementia often retain superficial social skills and can employ them even if they don't have full understanding of a situation. It will be helpful to Bob if Ron introduces himself and the purpose of his visit: 'Hello Bob, it's Ron; we used to play bowls together. I've come to see you to have a chat and see how you're getting on.' This helps Bob attend to the conversation more effectively.

- Ron's voice should be clear, but not too loud. He should keep the conversation simple and specific. He should use reflection to acknowledge Bob's contributions to the conversation. If Bob's responses to what he says contain unreal beliefs or 'confused' speech, Ron should try some of the responses discussed above.

## ASKING A PERSON WITH DEMENTIA QUESTIONS

Some people suggest that a person with dementia shouldn't be asked questions as they may have difficulty finding an appropriate answer and become distressed as a result. We would not go as far as this. Research indicates that people whose dementia has progressed certainly can answer questions and express their views on a range of topics. It is important that they are enabled as much as possible to make choices about aspects of their lives, and asking them questions is normally necessary for them to exercise choice.

At the same time, it is important to ask people with dementia questions in a way that they can answer. As suggested above, it is very easy to overestimate the person's cognitive abilities. Anything other than the most straightforward question may, indeed, be too difficult for the person. Asking them about aspects of their past lives is unlikely to gain more than a perfunctory response. Questions should be set in the here-and-now and framed in such a way that the person can use the information to hand in order to make a reply. Even a question such as 'What would you like to drink?' or 'Which dress would you like to wear today?' may be too hard for the person, as they may not remember the range of possible options. Framing such questions in the form 'Would you like tea or coffee?' or 'Would you like to wear this dress or that dress?' (whilst showing the person the dresses) allows the person to make choices.

## GUIDING AND INSTRUCTING

People whose dementia has progressed can retain some independence in daily living skills such as washing, dressing, going to the toilet and eating and drinking, but may need some help and guidance to do so. Similarly, as we discuss below, they can take part in activities but, again, may need assistance and direction. What communication skills do family members and friends need in order to assist those whose dementia has progressed to remain independent and active? Broadly speaking, we will need to give them instructions and guidance. The following are some basic principles that may be useful:

- Begin by orientating the person to the task or activity, even if it is one that is very familiar: 'It's eight o'clock Mum, I'm going to help you get dressed now.' It may be that the person will need to be re-orientated at times during the activity.

- Remember that the person may not be able to comprehend abstract ideas, or even familiar things that are not in their field of view. Complement your verbal instructions by showing the person the dress you are going to help them put on, or the cup you are going to put their drink into. The person may not remember where the kitchen is, and when taking them there it may be helpful to break down the journey into stages: 'We're going through the door here into the hall' (pointing towards the door); 'We're just turning into this room here' (pointing the way again).

- Breaking a task down into its constituent parts and slowly talking through the various stages will help overcome executive function issues. Keeping a flow of instructions will help the person attend and remain orientated.

- Sometimes the person will not at first understand or respond to even simple instructions. It is easy for family members or friends to get frustrated with the person, and even angry when this happens. It is important not to do so as the person will pick up on that frustration and may become more alarmed and agitated as a consequence. A good approach in this situation is to calmly repeat the instruction, perhaps wording it in a slightly different way. If the person still does not respond, wait a second or two and repeat again. It may take a few goes, but the person will usually pick up the message before too long.

Human activity is governed by communication and language, and by using simple principles such as those above, family and friends can help the person retain as much choice and independence as possible and maximise their sense of well-being.

## MAINTAINING INDEPENDENCE AS DEMENTIA PROGRESSES

As well as continuing relationships and interaction with the person, it is also important to help them maintain a degree of independence, at least within their own home. The following ideas may be helpful in achieving this aim:

- *Labelling and signage:* Signage can help the person find their way around the home if they no longer recognise some of the rooms or cupboards. You can use sticky labels or print signs for sticking on cupboards to indicate how to find items like cutlery, plates and food items. Using images as well as words and keeping things at eye level will help the person maintain independence. Examples of these can also be found on some internet sites providing assistive aids for people with dementia (see the Resources section at the end of the book).

- *Adaptations and removing clutter:* Some adaptations can make things easier to use and will help someone in carrying out an activity. Products such as jar openers or dementia-friendly crockery and utensils, which have a colour contrast on the rim, can be found on disability aid internet sites. It may also be helpful to ask for an assessment from an occupational therapist who will be able to offer advice. Keeping out only the things that are necessary for a task and having regular clear-outs will also be helpful.

- *Memory aids and instructions:* Providing prompts for someone to follow may help them feel less dependent on others and improve their sense of achievement. Try breaking down tasks into simple steps or writing simple reminders and instructions for someone to follow.

- *Light and noise:* Having adequate lighting is important in helping orientation and recognition. Try taking down any unnecessary curtains or blinds and increase the wattage on light bulbs. When doing activities, try to reduce noise from the television or radio, as this will help concentration.

- *Safety:* Ensuring the person is safe, especially if they are doing things alone, is important. The local fire service can be contacted to provide a free home safety check and advice regarding smoke alarms, which may be fitted free for people who are eligible. Other considerations include ensuring gas and electric appliances are checked regularly, and if you are concerned about people leaving things on, either isolation valves for gas cookers or cooker guards for electric cookers can be installed. Again, contact the occupational therapist for advice. Preventing falls is also an important consideration, and removing trip hazards such as loose rugs and objects on the floor is important. For people with visual difficulties, avoiding patterned or shiny flooring, if possible, will help them to find their way around.

- *Visual aids:* Making things easier to access and interpret will help someone maintain their independence. Try using a clock that includes a numerical time and day as this will help to orientate someone. Other suggestions to promote independence include having a plug-in night light to help someone find the bathroom at night, having a toilet seat that is a contrasting colour to the rest of the bathroom, and using cutlery and plates that are easy to recognise and use. Examples of all of these can be found on assistive aid sites designed for people with dementia.

- *Adapting clothing:* If someone is struggling with coordination and/or getting dressed, it may be helpful to simplify their clothing. For example, having trousers or tops that don't require buttons can make it easier for someone to dress themselves or for you to help them.

- *Reducing overstimulation:* Having too many noises or sounds at once can be overwhelming and cause either distress or withdrawal. Try to avoid having too many sights and sounds going on at once, reduce unnecessary background noise, and choose one activity at a time.

# CHAPTER 7

# Social and Leisure Activities as Dementia Progresses

In Chapter 5 we considered how to help people remain active in early dementia. We made the point that many people can, with assistance, maintain some or all of the activities that they enjoyed prior to developing dementia. As dementia progresses, however, the person's developing cognitive difficulties will affect their ability to engage in their accustomed activities.

> 'So after doing some artwork in day care, he would come home and would tear up his painting and throw it in the bin. He had problems with his visual-spatial awareness; the upper left side was all blank, and so the painting was just all down the right side and along the bottom. He knew it was rubbish and he came home in a worse temper than when he went there.' (Family member)

Some things will have to be given up and others will need to be adapted for the person to be able to take part in them. It may also be that the person responds better to activities they have not previously been used to doing. The role of family members and friends (and professionals) becomes more important in helping a person remain active as dementia progresses.

The range of activities that people with dementia can engage with is very wide. However, family members and friends will need imagination and skill in order to help the person gain satisfaction and well-being from taking part. We also need to be careful that activities are relevant for that person, and sensitive to their changing abilities.

Many activities can be done within the home (or in a residential care setting), whilst some involve going out. Some activities that are well received by people with dementia may not seem appropriate for most older people, such as throwing and catching a ball. Some can be done by the person on their own, but others need to involve other people. Several might also need to be simplified for a person with dementia to be able to take part. Finally, some, such as housework or washing up, are not really social or leisure-based, but they are activities that the person may have been used to doing in the past and can still gain satisfaction from helping others. We now group the range of activities into broad headings and consider each in turn:

- *Going out:* activities that involve the person (with the assistance of others) going to places and doing things outside the place they live.

- *Helping out:* activities in which the person does things for others, or helps out around the house.

- *Exercising:* activities that involve physical exercise.

- *Activities of daily living:* this includes all aspects of the person meeting their own care needs, such as washing, dressing, eating and drinking.

- *Sights and sounds:* watching television or videos; listening to music or the radio.

- *Pastimes:* embracing hobbies, interests and games, including dolls and toys.

## GOING OUT

In Chapter 5 we encouraged family members and friends to support a person with early dementia to go out and socialise. As dementia progresses this may become more challenging.

The person's conversational skills may be impaired and other aspects of their social abilities may also be damaged, possibly leading to embarrassing situations. The person may lack awareness of where they are or where they are going and may need assistance to maintain safety. They may be experiencing difficulties using the toilet (see Chapter 8). Also, the person's memory and attention may be impaired to the point where they can only concentrate for a brief period of time. Given all these challenges, family, friends and professional carers may feel that taking a person whose dementia has progressed out of their usual living setting is 'too hard'.

It would be a shame, however, if this view prevailed. 'Trips out' are good for people with dementia, as they are good for the rest of us. There are, however, two key principles when taking a person with dementia out:

- *Don't be too ambitious:* Short, simple excursions are most likely to be successful. The person's memory and attention difficulties may mean that they are unlikely to be able to appreciate long or intellectually complex outings and may tire easily. For example, a person may have enjoyed visiting museums or going to sports matches, but as dementia progresses, this may need to be adapted to shorter visits. A short walk, a visit to a public garden, a brief church service or a quick visit to a pub or cafe are more likely to be appreciated by the person, particularly if those accompanying them engage them in conversation and point out interesting aspects of their surroundings.

- *Be prepared:* Planning the trip beforehand will help to make it a success, as will taking with you things that the person may need, particularly regarding using the toilet. Anticipating any issues that the person's behaviour may cause others is also important (see Chapter 8), but family and friends should not be put off by the possibility of the person not always 'keeping up appearances', so long as others are not too inconvenienced.

## HELPING OUT

Many people with dementia will in the past have spent a lot of their time and gained satisfaction and well-being from doing things around the house, such as cooking, cleaning, gardening and DIY, or doing things for others. As dementia progresses, they may lose the ability to cook a full meal or decorate a room or keep their garden in pristine condition. Some will also lose interest in such activities, but others will want to continue to help out, and family members and friends should look for ways of supporting them to continue to do so.

To achieve this, we must use empathy and creativity to find things that the person can do that are within their capabilities. Trial and error may be involved here. People with dementia engage better with activities that they can understand and respond to, and this often means simple and straightforward things. For example, a person who likes cooking may be able to help cut up vegetables, or decorate an iced cake with sweets. Someone who enjoyed housework could assist with dusting or washing up, and a keen gardener may enjoy deadheading flowers or watering plants. The person may need assistance and supervision even with such simple tasks, and family and friends should not expect perfect results – the activity is more important than the finished product.

'Dad gradually took over the cooking but he would sit mum at the kitchen table and let her do things so she felt like she was taking a lead.' (Family member)

'I think it's important that my husband still feels that he is part of our routine. For example, he always gets up before me and sets the table. He doesn't always get it right, but I still let him do it.' (Family member)

## EXERCISING

We have mentioned previously the importance of physical exercise for people with dementia. Exercise is good for the person's physical health; it may slow the progression of the condition and can help reduce restlessness and sleep disturbances. If the person has been used to taking exercise, they are likely to want to continue to do so, and even if the person has not valued exercise in the past, the benefits outlined above will hopefully encourage family members and friends to support the person with getting some exercise.

Walking is perhaps the best form of exercise for an older person with dementia, as mentioned above. Even a short walk around the neighbourhood done regularly will be beneficial to the person. Some people with dementia appear to have a considerable need to walk around; this is sometimes referred to as 'wandering', but it is more helpful to think of this as 'purposeful walking', which can be channelled in a positive way (discussed in Chapter 8). Other forms of exercise may be possible, such as visiting a swimming baths or playing bowls.

Within the home there are other opportunities for physical activity, taking into account both the person's cognitive and physical abilities. The person may enjoy simple aerobic exercises or yoga, or spending time on an exercise bike. Ball games such as carpet bowls or simple games of catch will be within the person's capabilities and can be surprisingly enjoyable!

## Adapting exercise

Many older people with dementia will have other health conditions as well as their dementia, so any form of exercise needs to be within their limitations. Consider how an activity might be changed slightly to make it easier for someone, for example doing aerobics from sitting – 'chair aerobics' – and make sure that instructions are simple. If you have any concerns about mobility or risk of falls, you can request an assessment from a physiotherapist who may also be able to suggest some suitable exercises.

## Social engagement

Some people are more likely to do something if it is part of a group as they will be encouraged to join in. Try finding local walking groups for people with dementia or local day centres or community groups that offer appropriate physical activities that the person might be interested in.

## ACTIVITIES OF DAILY LIVING

A person with dementia is likely to need more assistance with daily living activities such as washing and bathing, dressing, eating and drinking as their condition progresses. Those caring for the person, both family members and professional home or residential care staff, may regard providing such assistance as a chore or a task to be completed as quickly and efficiently as possible. Often this means doing for the person things that they could do for themselves, given enough time and appropriate help. It is our view that it is better if people with dementia are encouraged to meet as many of their daily living needs themselves as is possible. For many of us, activities of daily living are more than chores; they are enjoyable aspects of our lives. We like to choose what to wear and to get ourselves looking our best. We may enjoy relaxing in a bath and we look forward to mealtimes and drinks. People with dementia enjoy these things too.

To assist with this, empathy is again needed. Activities of daily living such as getting dressed make demands on the person's 'executive function' abilities as they involve decision-making and doing things in sequence. Those caring for the person should take steps to simplify tasks for the person. We have discussed above how the person could be assisted in choosing what to wear. Executive function difficulties can lead to the person getting muddled when dressing themselves, so laying out clothes in the order that the person needs to put them on, or handing the person items one after the other, will help them dress themselves appropriately. Similar assistance could be provided with washing, doing hair, make-up and jewellery, if the person wants to wear it. If someone is struggling with coordination when getting dressed, it may be helpful to simplify their clothing.

'One morning my dad put a patterned skirt with a flowered blouse on mum which didn't go – my mum would never have worn anything like that, and she went mad. She just looked at me, and if she could have, she'd have said, "Don't take me out looking like a fool." Dad didn't know what to do, so I sorted her wardrobe out into colour coordinations for him.' (Family member)

The same principles of helping the person make realistic choices and assisting them to maintain independence can also be applied to mealtimes. These can also be opportunities for conversation and socialising. By the way, we are not averse to people with dementia drinking alcohol if that is what they have been used to – within recommended limits, of course! We will discuss eating and drinking further in Chapter 8.

Another principle is to make allowances for the person not getting everything right and not to blame them if they make mistakes with dressing or have imperfect table manners. Our approach should be to tactfully help them along the right path.

## SIGHTS AND SOUNDS
### Television

Many people with dementia will have enjoyed watching television throughout their lives. For some, it would have been their main form of relaxation. To what extent can television watching continue to be an enjoyable pastime for people whose dementia has progressed?

Television programmes (and speech programmes on the radio) place considerable cognitive demands on the person, and many of them may be too difficult to follow. They demand memory, to follow plots and recognise characters. They are usually verbal in nature, placing demands on language skills.

Images change rapidly, making it hard for the person to keep up. It is not uncommon for people to misinterpret the images as being real, which may cause distress. Television programmes are also long when compared to the attention span of a person with dementia. Small wonder that before too long the person has either fallen asleep or got up and walked off when left to watch the television.

Television viewing can, however, be an enjoyable activity for people with dementia, if those caring for the person use it creatively. First, technology developments have led to the possibility of creating 'bespoke' programmes for the person. Videos could be made of the person's family or friends, places that the person knows and likes, or activities that the person particularly enjoys. If such videos are clear, simple and short, the person may gain great enjoyment from watching them. One such video can be shown to the person many times, and it is best if family members or friends can sit with the person and help them enjoy the video more by talking with them about the people and scenes as they appear in the 'programme'.

Another aspect of television watching is that family members and friends may be surprised by the kind of programme that the person may enjoy. The late University of Oxford Professor of Philosophy and novelist Iris Murdoch developed dementia in her early 70s, and was cared for by her husband John Bayley, himself a professor at Oxford. In his book *Iris*, Bayley describes sitting on the sofa with his wife watching *Teletubbies*, a television programme aimed at an audience of toddlers. As her condition progressed, Iris enjoyed *Teletubbies* and other children's programmes including cartoons and, as Bayley put it, watched them with 'something approaching glee'.

Programmes such as *Teletubbies* are simple and repetitive, contain few words and, importantly, are made up of bright, clear, colourful and straightforward images. People with dementia may be attracted to such programmes as they are easy for them to understand and relate to. Enjoyment of such programmes does not mean that the person is 'going back to childhood'. Like the rest of us, they are simply gaining stimulation and enjoyment from watching and listening to something they can follow.

We are not suggesting that all people with dementia should watch children's programmes. Sitting the person in front of CBeebies is likely to be as counter-productive as any other form of marathon television viewing. Everyone is different, and some will relate to particular programmes more than others. We would suggest, however, that family members and friends think more flexibly about what the person may appreciate and enjoy, and not dismiss programmes or activities aimed at young children.

## Music

Music is an important aspect of many people's lives, and again, people with dementia are no exception. Research has shown the extent that music can enhance the well-being of people with dementia. It may help reduce distress through relaxing the person and giving them something enjoyable to listen to. It has often been noted that people with dementia may be able to sing along to the lyrics of songs that they know well, even when in other respects their memory and language difficulties are quite marked. This seems to be due to the way the brain accesses music and associated emotional memories.

There are many ways that family members and friends may help a person with dementia enjoy music. Playing music during the day that the person likes is the most straightforward means of achieving this aim, although as with most of us, before too long music will seem to fade into the background and the person will stop attending to it. At the same time, relaxing background music can engender a good mood in the person.

Family members and friends may wish to make a shared activity out of music by sitting with the person and listening to particular pieces with them. Perhaps the person could be encouraged to sing along. If the person played a musical instrument, they could be assisted to continue to play, although they may well not have the ability they used to. Some people like playing simple percussion instruments such as drums and tambourines. Simple 'sing-along' songs often go down well. By this we mean songs that the person may have sung at school or in organisations such as churches or community groups. Songs and music from a younger age that have been listened to frequently also seem to be recalled more easily and can evoke positive feelings.

In order to encourage engagement and response, music is more likely to be of benefit if it is relevant to the person's preferences. We all, no doubt, have favourite pieces of music or songs that make us feel happy or sad but that are important to how we feel. Approaches such as 'music therapy' that use classical or orchestral pieces are also being increasingly recognised as being of benefit. For people living with dementia the use of music does seem to have a particularly significant role in supporting well-being, and as such can be a very important activity, especially as the person's abilities decline.

At the same time, we must recognise that the old are, as it were, getting younger – it won't be long before a generation of older people will come along that was brought up on Heavy Metal or Punk Rock – posing new challenges for those caring for them!

## PASTIMES

Perhaps all other activities that don't fit into one of the above categories may be grouped together under the heading of *pastimes*. This embraces all the hobbies, games and interests that the person enjoyed before they developed dementia. It may also include activities that are more often associated with childhood, such as dolls and toys. All the benefits of activity can be applied to the category of pastimes, and family and friends can again enhance the well-being of the person by assisting them in enjoying the activities.

At the same time, we must again remember to make allowances for the progression of dementia. Some pastimes that the person enjoyed in the past may now be too difficult to carry out. Card games, crosswords, quizzes, hobbies that involve making things or sports with complex rules may become difficult and will at least need to be adapted. For example, a person who enjoyed bowls may lose the ability to understand a match and the tactics involved. The person may still, however, be able to deliver a bowl accurately, and so a simplified game could be played where the aim is just to get a single bowl nearest to the 'jack'. In the same vein, simpler games could be substituted for more complex ones – a person who previously enjoyed Bridge may still be able to play Snap. We have mentioned previously how people with dementia may be assisted to help out with such activities as gardening and cooking by carrying out simple components of those activities, and the same may be applied to pastimes. For example, a person who previously knitted sweaters may be able to knit simple squares, and a keen painter could still use colours and make patterns. As ever, family members and friends need to be flexible, creative and non-blaming – the pastime is more important than its outcome or product. Sensitivity is required to make sure that the person does not become frustrated by not being able to carry out an activity with the same skill they used to. And, of course, we should not make the person carry out an activity they do not enjoy.

'When the Bingo apparatus came out at the day centre, my husband would make for the door at 100 miles an hour and the person in charge would say to me, like a head teacher to a parent, "He has been a bit difficult today." If I knew then what I know now, I would say, "Are you surprised, given the sort of activity you make him do?"' (Family member)

Another aspect of pastimes that people with dementia often enjoy is access to pets and other animals. Many will have been used to having pets, and those caring for them may be able to help them continue to look after and gain pleasure from dogs, cats and other animals. If keeping a pet is not possible, family members and friends can enhance the person's well-being by bringing their own pets to visit the person.

As well as animals, many people with dementia enjoy the company of children and babies, and family members and friends should not be afraid of bringing their children to visit the person, although often short well-supervised visits may be better for the person and for the child.

## Dolls and toys

We have discussed above ways that the person's accustomed pastimes may be adapted to take account of the progression of dementia and allow them to continue to enjoy those pastimes. There is a further aspect of pastimes that may be appropriate. This is the use of dolls, toys or children's games as ways of promoting activity with people with dementia. It is a controversial area, but research indicates that people with dementia may derive considerable well-being from dolls or children's toys.

Dolls, particularly life-like ones, are often much appreciated by people with dementia. Some will 'adopt' a doll as if it were their own child, and will take it around with them and look after it. Is this a good thing? Our view is that we see nothing wrong in a person with dementia deriving well-being in this way. It will do the person no harm, and 'looking after' a doll has the particular benefit of helping the person feel useful to another – something that in the 'real world' is denied them, due to their own dependence on others. Life-like toy dogs and cats can also enhance well-being in the same way.

Some have gone further and used a wide range of children's toys as a means of promoting activity with people with dementia. The range of electronic dolls and toys that is now available are particularly useful. A recent research project about the introduction of a robotic toy seal (called 'Paro') that responds to being touched or stroked by making noises or fluttering its eyes has produced remarkable results in terms of improving mood and increasing interaction in people with dementia. Other activities such as motorised cars and trains may go down well and have the benefit of supporting reminiscence. Enjoyment can also be gained from such things as balloons and bubbles and dressing up.

What do we make of the use of children's toys and games with people with dementia? The issues are the same as those in the example we gave above of Iris Murdoch watching *Teletubbies*. Dolls and children's toys are bright, simple and understandable to people with dementia. We ourselves have been surprised by the enthusiasm with which many people with dementia embrace dolls and toys, and have had to modify our own feelings of discomfort when using them – again, the proof of the pudding is in the eating, and whatever promotes enjoyment and well-being can't be bad.

## SUMMARY: PRINCIPLES OF PROMOTING ACTIVITY WITH PEOPLE WITH DEMENTIA

- *Anything a person with dementia does is an activity:* Our definition of activity is a broad one, embracing daily living activities as well as pastimes and 'passive' activities such as watching television. The trick is to make whatever the person does an opportunity to promote engagement with others and enhance well-being.

- *Make time for activities:* It is easy to regard activities as an 'optional extra', to be done only if possible. Our view is that activities are integral to the well-being of the person, and there is good evidence that people with dementia who are encouraged to be active are more engaged and experience less distress.

- *Be prepared to participate:* People whose dementia has progressed may have more difficulty in initiating activities and are likely to need assistance in carrying them out. Family members and friends should be prepared to participate in activities with the person and to take the lead.

- *Base activities on what the person has always liked to do:* Familiar activities are most likely to be enjoyed and the person may be better able to carry out activities they have been used to doing.

- *Use empathy and creativity to make activities achievable:* Activities need to be adapted, simplified and often shortened for people with dementia.

- *Make activities social occasions:* Take part in the activity yourself and encourage others to spend time with the person as well. Use activity times as opportunities for interaction and conversation.

- *Encourage independence and choices:* Let the person choose activities or aspects of an activity as much as possible, and allow the person to do as much for themselves as they can.

- *Remember safety:* It is important to ensure that the person is safe, especially if they are doing things alone (see Chapter 6).

- *Remember that the activity itself is more important than the outcome:* It is not important if the painting that the person produces or the cake they ice is not perfect. It is the fact that the person is experiencing well-being through being active that is key.

- *Consider dolls and toys:* The value of dolls, toys and children's games for promoting well-being in people with dementia is well established by research and the experience of many carers. If we can move beyond our reservations, we may find that the person will benefit from such things to a much greater extent than we think they will.

- *Ask for help and involve others:* For family carers who are doing a lot of the caring, it is important to ask others for help and support with activities, as this is an ideal way in which others can get involved and provide a valuable break. Equally for those who are less involved, it is really helpful to suggest an activity you can do with the person, as the main carer may find it difficult to ask for help.

# CHAPTER 8

# The Challenges of Dementia

There are a number of challenges that people living with dementia and their families and friends may face as dementia progresses. These can be caused by physical changes as a result of dementia or changes in comprehension, behaviour and ways of coping. Some changes can be particularly upsetting for family and friends who are supporting the person, and we address these under the broad heading of 'Changes in behaviour'. In addition, specific attention is given to the challenges of eating and drinking, using the toilet, sleeping and the potential difficulties of admission into hospital. Finally, we consider the sensitive issue of vulnerability and abuse.

## CHANGES IN BEHAVIOUR

We chose the heading for this section with care. We wish to avoid terms sometimes found in books for families or professional carers such as 'behaviour problems' or 'challenging behaviour'. Such terms seem to imply that the difficulty is with the person with dementia, that they are somehow doing something wrong or are in some way to blame for their behaviour. As described in Chapter 1, the various difficulties that someone with dementia can experience with memory, communication, cognitive abilities (thinking and processing), emotion or manner and physical changes can understandably lead to changes in their behaviour, including distress, agitation, withdrawal, disinhibition or being seemingly uncooperative.

> 'I do get angry if something does not work as it should – could be tying a shoelace or looking for a screwdriver. I also get annoyed when people don't speak clearly enough for me to understand, with the result that I withdraw from communication.' (Person with dementia)

When family members and friends feel challenged by the person's manner or actions, it is important for them to remember that the person may intend something very different by those actions to how it comes across to others. In other words, it isn't that the person is being 'challenging' or 'problematic'; the person is simply trying to relate to their world. At the same time, there is no doubt that *others* may find the person's behaviour challenging and may experience considerable feelings of stress as a result. Coping with such behaviour is a major issue for family members and friends of people with dementia. However, significant caution should be observed if there is a *sudden* increase in such things as agitated or distressed behaviour. Such changes may be as a result of a physical health issue such as an infection, constipation or dehydration, or a change in the person's medication. This may lead to the person experiencing *delirium* (see Chapter 3), and this should be ruled out and treated, if found to be the cause.

## What causes people with dementia to behave in ways that others find challenging?

We can offer two possible broad explanations that may underlie such changes in behaviour.

### The person's behaviour is a symptom of dementia

It used to be thought that most 'challenging behaviour' was a symptom of dementia. As we saw in Chapter 3, some types of dementia such as behavioural variant fronto-temporal dementia affect areas of the brain particularly associated with changes in emotion, manner and behaviour, leading to increased likelihood of the person behaving in socially inappropriate or puzzling ways. Equally, if someone is experiencing hallucinations as a result of dementia with Lewy bodies, or is having difficulty with interpreting their environment due to visual-perceptual difficulties, this may cause significant distress. As we have seen, awareness or comprehension may also be impaired for many people with dementia as the condition progresses, and similarly, awareness of the consequences of behaviour may not be recognised.

### The person is trying to get their needs met

Research is increasingly showing that much of the behaviour that others find challenging is as a result of unmet needs which, because of their condition, the person cannot express or meet themselves. Sometimes the need is an immediate one; for example, a person may become agitated because they need the toilet or are in pain. Sometimes the need reflects aspects of the person's life history, such as a person who lived on a farm wanting to be outdoors. Family members and friends can use their knowledge of the person to identify the underlying need and help the person get their needs met. Our view is that we should always assume that the person's manner and actions are meaningful, rather than that the person's behaviour is random or a symptom of their dementia. Only if it is clear that no meaning can be found in the person's behaviour should other explanations be sought.

'My husband used to shake his fist and swear at himself in the mirror. Years later I understood what was going on. He couldn't recognise himself because, with recent memories erased, he thought he was a young man again, and also, because of visual-spatial problems, he thought the reflection was a real person. He was thinking: "Who is this stranger in my house?" Maybe he thought, "My wife is being unfaithful."' (Family member)

## How should we respond to behaviour that we find challenging?

To an extent, our answer to this question will depend on what we feel to be the cause of the behaviour. If we feel it is simply a symptom of dementia, we might be inclined to look for medical responses such as medication. Alternatively, if we attribute behaviour to the person attempting to get their needs met, we might be more inclined to use psychological strategies to find the underlying need and to assist the person to meet that need. If the need is for psychological comfort and well-being, then approaches such as reminiscence, music and aromatherapy may be appropriate (see the Resources section at the end of the book for further information). We discuss the role of medication below, but in general, psychological approaches should always be used first. In this section we look more closely at those aspects of behaviour that family and friends find challenging, and suggest some simple ways that we might respond.

### What aspects of behaviour do family and friends find challenging?

Broadly speaking, we can identify a number of categories of behaviour that family and friends find challenging. These overlap somewhat, and a person's behaviour may sometimes fall into several of the categories:

- When the person lacks awareness that their actions will put them at risk of harm

- When the person's manner and actions indicate that they are in distress

- When the person appears to be apathetic or unmotivated

- When the person behaves in ways that are considered socially inappropriate

- When the person seems to be unwilling to accept help from others, and their basic needs such as eating and drinking or using the toilet are compromised

- When the person tries to get their needs met through behaving aggressively or with hostility.

We explore these categories in more detail below.

### WHEN THE PERSON LACKS AWARENESS THAT THEIR ACTIONS WILL PUT THEM AT RISK OF COMING TO HARM

We discussed in Chapter 5 how a person with dementia might, through trying to carry on with their accustomed lives, put themselves at risk of harm. As dementia progresses, such risks may diminish if the person's declining abilities and awareness mean that such independent actions occur less. However, that decline in abilities and awareness carries its own risks as the person becomes more and more reliant on others. One aspect of risk is that of abuse or exploitation by others, which we consider later.

One of the 'risky behaviours' that family members and friends are most often concerned about is when the person has a profound need to be on their feet and to walk about, but lacks awareness of where they are or how to get from one place to another – and more importantly, how to get back safely. As we have seen, such walking about is often called 'wandering', but we dislike this term as it implies aimlessness. Instead, we would use the term *purposeful walking* as the person is likely to be fulfilling an inner need or purpose. The need may be related to their current situation: perhaps the person is experiencing pain or discomfort. Often walking about derives from boredom, if the person's day is empty. Sometimes the person simply wants some exercise. If the period of walking is prolonged, it could be that the person has forgotten how long they have been on their feet.

It is worth mentioning a phenomenon known as *sundowning* here, which is a term used to describe changes in behaviour that commonly occur in the evening, around dusk. It is often associated with people with dementia having a strong need to go out or walk around as they may feel they are in the wrong place. There are lots of reasons why this happens, but it can be due to people becoming more disorientated due to tiredness, or being hungry, thirsty or in pain.

Other explanations for walking about may derive from the person's life history. We mentioned above a farmer who was always used to being outside. The person may have had a job that involved being on their feet, or recreational walking may have always been an important part of their life.

The chief risk associated with walking about is the possibility of the person getting lost. An associated risk is that the person may fall, especially if they are becoming physically frail. If the person wants to go outdoors, they may become frustrated if they cannot do so and become agitated as a consequence, thereby compounding the difficulty experienced by those caring for the person.

How should we respond when the person displays such behaviour? As the person has a clear need to walk about, we should find ways for the person to do so safely rather than preventing them from being active. Ideally, family members and friends will find time to go out for walks with the person – as we saw earlier, exercise is good for all people with dementia. If the person's main carer is less physically active, then other family members or friends could perhaps go out with them. Providing activities during the day and involving the person in what is going on may reduce boredom. If the person was previously less active, investigations for pain or other possible physical causes of restlessness should be carried out. Steps could be taken to allow the person to walk about indoors safely by clearing ways and removing obstacles that the person could fall over. If it is the evening, as described in 'sundowning', strategies such as closing the curtains before dusk, limiting caffeinated drinks and doing a relaxing activity together may help reduce distress. Activities such as playing relaxing music or using aromatherapy are recommended as beneficial approaches.

What if the person is insistent on going outside when it is not possible for someone to go with them? Increasingly, assistive technology is playing a role in keeping people safe whilst allowing them freedom to walk outside, through devices that individuals carry on their person. These devices, which are available in various forms such as mobile phones, pendants, key ring attachments and shoe inserts, act as a tracking system using GPS, which allows others to find out where the person is. Alternatively, a simpler option may be to have a label or necklace on the person that provides emergency information should the person get lost.

For those who are considered unsafe to go out alone, some would resort to locking the door (making sure it could be opened quickly in an emergency, such as a fire). This may be sufficient to put the person off, but some may become more upset and frustrated as they try in vain to open the door, and more creative approaches may be needed. Perhaps it is possible for the person to go into the garden on their own, if the gate to the road is locked. Sometimes it is possible to disguise the door so that the person does not realise where it is. These are drastic measures, but those caring for the person may perhaps be excused for putting safety first.

At present there are no legal ramifications for such measures if they are in the person's best interests and to ensure their safety. However, legislation based on the Deprivation of Liberty Safeguards (DoLS) that currently apply to care homes and hospitals (see Chapter 9) is being prepared to provide a legal underpinning to the protection of people living in the community who lack capacity. The new legislation will be known as Liberty Protection Safeguards (LPS).

### WHEN THE PERSON'S MANNER AND ACTIONS INDICATE THAT THEY ARE IN DISTRESS

People whose dementia has progressed can experience the full range of emotions, but sometimes due to their processing and language difficulties they are not able to clearly express how they are feeling. Their emotions may, however, be reflected in their behaviour. It is always worth considering if the person might be in pain or physically unwell, yet unable to express this. It is not uncommon for older people in particular to have other conditions that cause them discomfort such as arthritis, gastric problems or dental pain. If the person is distressed, it is important to establish if there is a physical cause so that this can be treated. However, if this proves difficult, offering mild pain relief and observing its effect is worth a try.

> 'Find out the cause and address this first. Other things that might help include engaging me in conversation, distract me and show me happy photos.' (Person with dementia)

Whilst walking about may be a sign of boredom, it could also be that the person is feeling anxious, perhaps half remembering events from the past and believing that they should be doing something. Anxiety is a not uncommon feeling amongst people with dementia. As their awareness declines, the world can become a confusing and even frightening place as they become increasingly unable to understand what is happening to them or what is going on around them. Anxiety may manifest itself in the person becoming restless and agitated, asking questions over and over and continually seeking the presence and reassurance of familiar people. Family members and friends may understandably find such behaviour tiring and frustrating.

> 'My husband became quite anxious, partly because I became crosser with him. I would say: "You have just asked me that – you've asked me that eight times today." I am not a very patient person.' (Family member)

Restlessness may also result from the environment that the person is living in. We have discussed previously that the person's attention difficulties will make noisy and overactive environments stressful. If the person does not understand where they are or how to find places such as the toilet, anxiety may again be increased.

Anxiety may also be a consequence of the person experiencing symptoms such as hallucinations or delusions or misinterpreting their environment. These may cause the person distress if the perception or belief is unpleasant, sad or frightening.

It is important that those caring for the person use empathy to try to appreciate why the person is feeling the way they do. Difficult though it can sometimes be, try to remain calm and reassuring – if we show our anger or frustration, it will almost certainly increase the person's anxiety. If you find yourself getting angry or frustrated, try walking into another room and taking some deep breaths before returning. Spending quality time with the person, including them in what is going on and keeping them orientated by telling them what is happening on a regular basis may help reassure and calm the person.

'If I was distressed, I would want people to back off and give me space. Don't tell me anything that makes me think it's my fault. Please repeat things, but without any undertone of criticism.' (Person with dementia)

Another emotion that people with dementia may experience is depression. Research indicates that depression is at its most common during the middle years of dementia. The person may not be able to express their feelings verbally, but depression may result in them becoming upset and tearful, or may lead to them appearing to be withdrawn, unmotivated or apathetic. Alternatively, they may become more agitated and restless. The best way that family and friends can help is through giving the person time and love and encouraging them to do some activities – psychologists tell us that trying to stay active is one of the best medicines for those who are depressed. Psychological therapies or medication may be helpful if the person is profoundly depressed.

## WHEN THE PERSON APPEARS TO BE APATHETIC OR UNMOTIVATED

This is a frequent complaint of family members and friends. The person with dementia is reluctant to do things, preferring to sit and do nothing whilst those around them become frustrated at their perceived lack of motivation.

Once again, we must begin by challenging the use of terms. 'Apathy' and 'lack of motivation' are loaded expressions that imply criticism of the person or even an element of blame. Instead, we must again try to empathise with the person and find possible reasons why their levels of activity have reduced. There are many possibilities:

- They might be depressed and need psychological support or therapy.

- They may be feeling anxious. At some level the person may recognise their cognitive disabilities and be reluctant to put themselves into certain situations (including social situations) when they may feel they won't be able to cope.

- They may misunderstand what is being suggested to them. We might say something like: 'Come on Mum, it's time to go to the day centre.' But Mum may not remember going to the day centre or understand what a day centre is and might refuse to go, through wariness of the unknown.

- Their perception of the world may be changing. As dementia progresses, the person's ability to attend to and respond to the world will reduce, and they may be content to live largely within their own little sphere.

These possible explanations for a person's reduced activity levels suggest strategies for responding. Assessment and treatment of depression may be appropriate. Reassurance and a non-blaming approach may reduce anxiety, and clear and repeated explanations may help the person better understand suggested activities. But sometimes, family and friends have to come to terms with the fact that their loved one is changing, and that a reduction in activity is often simply a consequence of the person's increasing cognitive difficulties. Whilst we would not advocate leaving the person to sit doing nothing all day, sometimes we must accept reduced activity levels and a modification of activities to better meet the needs of the person.

'I think the thing we found hardest wasn't grandma forgetting things, but the lack of interest she has in life, the things she used to enjoy like going to garden centres; if you take her now she'll just walk behind you, she won't look around her and see what's there... The majority of the time grandma will just sit there and gaze into space, but I don't think she has the same awareness of time; she gets lost in her own head thinking about things, and I don't think it's as horrendous as others think.' (Family member)

### WHEN THE PERSON BEHAVES IN WAYS THAT ARE CONSIDERED SOCIALLY INAPPROPRIATE

Family members and friends can become very upset if the person's manner and actions are not socially appropriate – if they are rude, messy, untidy, over-talkative or disinhibited. Empathy with the person should again assure us this is not deliberate, but that such behaviour is a manifestation of loss of cognitive abilities. In particular, executive function impairment will affect the person's judgement in social situations. Up to a point, the best strategy is to make allowances for the person – as John Bayley put it in *Iris*, 'On no account try to keep up appearances.' Sometimes those caring for the person create problems for themselves by expecting too much of the person or by insisting that things should be as they were before the person developed dementia – it is understandable, though, that the family should wish that this was so.

At the same time, we are not suggesting that socially inappropriate behaviour should be totally ignored. For one thing, people with dementia do not want to be the way they are. If they could magically be cured of dementia and look back at the way they had been behaving, they may be shocked, embarrassed and upset. Family members and friends sometimes need to uphold the person's dignity by gently correcting or diverting them if they start to act in ways that upset others or would upset themselves if they knew what they were doing.

> 'I think a couple of our neighbours have found it quite difficult. My husband sometimes says things that are inappropriate due to the nature of his dementia and he must have said something rude to a neighbour. One day he [the neighbour] avoided us both in the street; he had previously ignored my husband but not me. So I wrote to him explaining the reason.' (Family member)

This particularly applies when, as sometimes happens, the person becomes sexually disinhibited and starts making inappropriate advances towards someone else (discussed in Chapter 5). In all cases it is important to maintain respect for the person and not to abandon them if they do not always act the way they used to.

WHEN THE PERSON SEEMS TO BE UNWILLING TO ACCEPT HELP FROM OTHERS
People with dementia often need considerable assistance with daily living activities, but may not always be willing to accept such assistance. As we have seen, they may resist when being helped to get washed and dressed or when those caring for them want them to go somewhere and may respond aggressively if pressed. This, not unnaturally, causes frustration in carers.

If such situations arise, we should again try to understand the situation from the person's perspective, to see if we can identify reasons for the person's resistance. It may be that the person was approached in the wrong way, or not given enough orientation to what the carer was intending to do and felt threatened and defensive as a result. Perhaps they did not recognise who was with them, even though it was someone very familiar to them, or perhaps they just didn't want to get dressed at that moment, thank you very much!

Those caring for the person can try a range of approaches when the person resists in this way. First and foremost, is it possible to respect the person's wishes not to be disturbed – do they have to get washed or dressed at that time?

> 'My husband went through a phase of not wanting to take off his jogging bottoms, and went to bed in them. So we had these scenes with me saying, "Come on, you have to take your trousers off before going to bed", but the outreach worker said, "There is no law against going to bed in your tracksuit bottoms" so suddenly, that problem disappeared, because someone told me how to deal with it – it was my problem, not his – just let it go.' (Family member)

Sometimes leaving the person and coming back later is all that is required. If the activity of daily living is necessary, trying to orientate the person as much as possible may help. This could involve a clear explanation of what is wanted, perhaps reinforced by visual cues, for example holding the person's dress up so they can see it. Involving the person in the activity and offering choices and opportunities for them to do things for themselves may enhance understanding. If the person does not appear to understand instructions, repeating those instructions calmly and clearly, perhaps changing the wording a little, may help the message get through. Another strategy might be to use distraction by playing music, singing along with the person or talking about a pleasurable activity.

> 'My husband was also whopping me one, so when the carer was washing him I was holding his hands and singing to him, talking to him and distracting him whilst the carer was getting on with the job. Then another carer came once a week to give him a bath. He disliked showers because he thought it was somebody hitting him, so he hit back.' (Family member)

WHEN THE PERSON TRIES TO GET THEIR NEEDS MET THROUGH
BEHAVING AGGRESSIVELY OR WITH HOSTILITY

Unsurprisingly, this is an aspect of dementia that causes particular stress for those caring for the person. Aggressive behaviour includes verbal threats, swearing and hostile utterances and physical aggression, such as hitting, slapping, spitting and scratching. It is fortunately rare that a person with dementia seriously injures another, but it can happen, particularly if they are being cared for by someone who is themselves an older person. Those with young-onset dementia can potentially cause more injury.

Sadly, aggression is a fact of everyday life. How often have we found ourselves being shouted at in a family row, been on the receiving end of an angry driver's blaring horn or had to manage an irate customer at work? How often have we been the ones dishing out the aggression in these situations? Most of us have the potential to act aggressively if we are threatened, frustrated or our needs are not being met. People with dementia are no different to the rest of us, but due to their condition, they may act aggressively in a wider range of situations than they would previously have done, due again to cognitive and language difficulties preventing them from getting their needs met in more appropriate ways.

Usually, aggressive behaviour happens in response to an outside event that acts as a *trigger*. Sometimes, family members and friends can themselves trigger aggression, if they approach the person in an angry or blaming way.

It may be that relationships within the family have always been volatile, with frequent arguments, and if these continue when the person develops dementia, then actual physical aggression may result. Interacting with a potentially aggressive person requires a calm and reassuring manner. The qualities of patience and acceptance are never more important than when the person is prone to acting aggressively.

> 'Suddenly it was much easier; I had been trying to take over but I suddenly realised that some of my husband's aggression was because I was being too bossy – "Come on, put your shoes on" – treating him like a child.' (Family member)

Aggression may result if the person is being helped to do something they don't want to do, or they don't understand the reason for. A common trigger for aggression is when others are trying to give personal care, such as helping the person wash or dress. Conversely, aggressive behaviour may arise if the person is being prevented from doing something that they wish to do, such as going outside when it is not convenient for them to do so. Aggression can result from the person not understanding their situation and feeling frightened and vulnerable. Understanding the underlying need that the aggressive person is expressing is the first step to making an appropriate response. However, if you feel you are at risk, it is always sensible to remove yourself from the situation for a short while, allowing the person to calm down and return after a short break.

## The role of medication

Whilst the interpersonal strategies discussed in this section (and summarised below) can help relations with a person with dementia considerably, there is no doubt that family members and friends can remain troubled by aspects of the person's behaviour, and those caring for the person can experience considerable stress as a result of the person's manner and actions. Research has shown that these issues are the main reasons why informal caring relationships break down and residential care is sought for the person. Despite the range of interpersonal approaches available to family members and friends for easing relationships with people with dementia, the person may still act in ways that cause difficulties, frustration and stress for those caring for them. In these circumstances desperate carers often see medication as being the answer and will appeal to their doctor to give the person 'something to calm them down'. GPs may be at a loss to suggest alternatives and can end up acquiescing to such requests.

Three broad types of medication are available that may make the person's manner and behaviour more manageable. First, there is some evidence that the AChE inhibitor drugs given to people in the early years of dementia (see Chapter 3) may help by making the person better orientated to their surroundings and therefore less prone to being resistant or defensive due to misunderstanding. Another drug called 'memantine' is available for people with more advanced dementia that is aimed at reducing occurrences of distressed behaviour. Current evidence is that the effects of all these drugs are modest. Recent research has suggested that mild painkillers given on a regular basis may be just as effective in easing distress, suggesting that much agitation and aggression may be due to the person experiencing pain or physical discomfort (although medical advice should be sought before these are given, due to potential side effects).

Second, anxiolytic drugs may sometimes be prescribed to attempt to treat anxiety, in particular drugs from the benzodiazepine group such as diazepam (Valium) or lorazepam (Ativan). However, caution is required when considering the use of these drugs as they are known to increase both the risk of falls and cognitive impairment, potentially making the situation worse. In most cases anxiety is a long-term feeling for people with dementia, and these drugs are ineffective and potentially harmful if given for more than a few weeks.

The third broad group of drugs that can be prescribed for people with dementia are 'antipsychotic' drugs, namely risperidone or haloperidol. In the UK these are only licensed for people with dementia who are at risk of harming themselves or others through experiencing agitation, hallucinations or delusions that are causing them severe distress. These drugs aim to reduce hallucinations and delusions and have a sedative effect to help reduce agitation and restlessness. They can have significant side effects including Parkinson-like symptoms (such as jerky movements, tremors or stiffness), headaches, changes in appetite, and feeling sleepy or less alert. The most serious side effect for those who are on these drugs for a long period is increased risk of stroke or even death. As such, these drugs should be used with caution, and only be prescribed for short periods and reviewed regularly.

'When my husband shouted and swore at his reflection he was given an antipsychotic; it increased his confusion and caused him to shuffle, and it brought on a mild heart attack, when all I should have done was take the mirrors down. Again, it was everyone's ignorance about what can trigger aggressive behaviour.' (Family member)

'I would be happy for occasional use of medication if it's needed but I do not want a "chemical cosh". I want to be in the conditions and surroundings where I can find calm and not get wound up.' (Person with dementia)

If given appropriately, antipsychotic medication may, on occasion, be a necessary and helpful option in providing a way of reducing distressing symptoms and avoiding breakdown in the caring situation.

'I was being aggressive towards my wife, and if it hadn't been for the fact I was given an antipsychotic which calmed me down, my wife would never have spoken to me again *or* continued supporting me. That would have been much worse than the risks of taking it!' (Person with dementia)

**Summary: how should family members and friends respond when they find the person's behaviour challenging?**

- Remember that the person almost certainly does not mean to be difficult. They are trying to fulfil a need they cannot express in a conventional way.

- Adopt a calm and reassuring approach. Don't argue with the person or raise your voice, even when you are feeling frustrated by their behaviour.

- Ensure that the person's environment is calming and orientating.

- Use empathy to try to ascertain the meaning behind the person's actions. What need are they trying to fulfil, and does it relate to their present circumstances or to their past life?

- Check that the person's behaviour is not due to pain or physical discomfort.

- Reduce the person's anxiety by including them in events. Try to keep them orientated to their surroundings and what is happening around them.

- Be flexible and tolerant. Find ways of allowing the person to walk about safely. Don't insist on the person doing things they are refusing to do, unless it is absolutely necessary.

- Involve the person in regular activities and exercise. It will relieve boredom, use up excess energy and may lift the person's mood.

- At the same time, recognise that the person's world is changing, and gear activities accordingly (see Chapter 7).

- Try alternative strategies such as music or aromatherapy to help ease the person's anxiety and improve their sense of well-being.

- Ask for medication only as a last resort, and don't expect too much from it. Look out for signs that the person is experiencing side effects.

## CHALLENGES TO EATING AND DRINKING

We all need to eat and drink and on the whole enjoy eating and drinking. People with dementia are no different, but as dementia progresses the person is likely to need assistance meeting their nutritional needs. In this section we consider how those caring for the person can help them eat a good diet and gain satisfaction from food and drink.

As the condition progresses, it is not uncommon for people with dementia to lose weight. It is often thought that weight loss is an inevitable part of the physical decline that accompanies advancing dementia. This is not, however, the case until perhaps the end of life stage, which will be considered in Chapter 11. Weight loss usually results from the person simply not eating or drinking enough. This can sometimes be due to poor understanding of the person's needs and preferences for food and drink and not ensuring they have an adequate intake. The consequences of low body weight can be serious as it increases the risk of a number of harmful conditions, including hypothermia, osteoporosis, fracture, depression, impaired immunity, delayed healing, pressure sores and micronutrient deficiencies.

For some people the problem may be overeating or inappropriate eating, such as eating too much of one type of food or trying to eat non-edible products due to poor recognition. Alternatively, it may be due to another problem such as an infection, constipation, ill-fitting dentures or oral thrush, all of which should be investigated and treated. If a person with dementia cannot meet their own nutritional needs as the condition progresses, carers must take on that responsibility themselves.

What is an appropriate diet for an older person with dementia? Overall, what is healthy for the rest of us is healthy for someone with dementia. However, it is generally better for older people to be slightly overweight than underweight, so if the person is experiencing weight loss, a diet high in calories may be appropriate. Plenty of bread, cakes, potatoes, sugar, fats and chocolate may not be recommended for most of us but are just the ticket for an older person who is losing weight! Those caring for the person should consult their GP, and advice from a dietician may be beneficial.

## Difficulties with eating and drinking

Dementia may affect the person's ability to meet their nutritional needs in a number of ways, and those caring for the person should again use empathy to appreciate why the person is having difficulties. Possible explanations for eating and drinking difficulties include:

- *Untreated pain or discomfort:* This is often overlooked as people may not have been able to have their teeth checked and may have untreated dental problems, mouth ulcers and/or ill-fitting dentures. Understandably this will make people reluctant to eat, and every effort should be made to treat any problems. Community dentists who are appropriately trained in understanding dementia may be required.

- *Impaired recognition of food and drink:* The person's memory and attention difficulties may lead them to simply not notice that food has been put in front of them, particularly if it has been placed beyond their immediate field of attention, or they may not recognise it as food. People with visual difficulties may have problems with differentiating between the plate, table and food.

- *Loss of ability to express likes, dislikes and preferences:* If the person is given a meal by someone who does not know them well, they may be given something they dislike, but may not be able to express their feelings clearly. Sometimes people with dementia come to dislike food that they previously enjoyed, perhaps due to their condition affecting their sense of taste.

- *Impaired ability to concentrate on a meal:* The person's memory and attention difficulties may make it hard for them to concentrate on a meal long enough to finish it. They may leave a meal half-eaten, and those caring for them will assume that they have had enough, but it could be that their attention has wandered. Sometimes a person who likes to walk about a lot may find it hard to sit still for long enough to eat a full meal.

- *Impaired ability to use cutlery:* Impairment of executive function can affect the person's ability to use a knife and fork with proper skill, or to cut up food. Again, this may result in the person leaving food due to them not being able to put it in their mouth successfully.

• *Impaired hand–mouth coordination:* The person's ability to coordinate fine movements such as putting food into their mouth may also be impaired. The person may drop food and not be able to retrieve it or may eat 'messily', becoming reluctant to finish their meal due to embarrassment.

## Helping a person with dementia meet their nutritional needs

As with other aspects of behaviour, understanding the reasons for that behaviour is the first step to finding creative solutions. In no particular order, we offer the following suggestions for helping the person eat and drink properly:

• *Know the person's accustomed eating habits:* Despite the possibility of tastes changing, most people will enjoy best those foods that they have always preferred. Maintaining accustomed routines is also important, so that the person eats at times and in a place they are used to.

• *Provide an environment conducive to eating and drinking:* A distraction-free and relaxing environment will help the person concentrate on their meal and will reduce restlessness. Clear lighting and a minimum of extraneous noise is helpful. It may be better to leave the television off, and have relaxing background music instead. Eating is often more pleasurable as a social occasion, so eat together or with others wherever possible.

• *Promote attention to food:* Food that is colourful and easily recognised is best. Ensure that the person knows that their meal is there by putting food and drink where they can see and recognise it, and tell them what it is. Having a contrast between the plate and the table is helpful for visual-spatial difficulties, for example having bright coloured plates against a plain different-coloured tablecloth or having a visible rim round the edge of the plate. Offer smaller portions and provide meals or snacks more frequently, as large portions may be too much for some people and put them off eating.

• *Encourage and assist as necessary – but don't patronise:* The person who has difficulties with using cutlery or with hand-to-mouth coordination may need some assistance with eating, but the principle should be to maintain the person's independence and dignity as much as possible. Adapted cutlery can be bought that helps people grip and coordinate better (see the Resources section, 'Disability aids for people with dementia'). The person should only be helped to eat if they really cannot manage themselves (see Chapter 10). Sometimes it will be appropriate to cut up the person's food so they can manage it better, or for the person to use a spoon rather than a knife and fork. Alternatively, the person may manage better with 'finger food' that they can pick up. As anyone who has organised a buffet party knows, there is a wide range of tasty foods that can be served to be eaten without cutlery!

• *Minimise constipation through high-fibre food, adequate hydration and promoting exercise:* Constipation is a frequent difficulty for people with dementia, and it may make them reluctant to eat or restless through discomfort. Constipation can be minimised by including high-fibre foods, particularly vegetables and fruit, in the person's diet, and by ensuring that they drink adequate fluids and by promoting exercise.

• *Adopt a flexible approach if the person cannot concentrate on meals:* Sometimes it is better to make food available on a flexible basis if the person is too restless to concentrate on set mealtimes. Offer frequent snacks and drinks during the day that can be eaten easily if the person is walking about. Sometimes the person will feel hungrier at night times, so making snacks available then may help settle them.

- *Monitor the person's weight:* Weight loss can be serious, so those caring for the person should keep the person's weight under review. Dementia does not in itself lead to weight loss, so if the person is losing weight, it is for another reason, as mentioned above. Also, people who walk about much of the time may lose weight due to the amount of exercise they are having. In these cases, bulking up meals with extra carbohydrates, fats and proteins may be appropriate. Weight loss may also reflect an underlying physical health problem that may require medical attention. Some people with dementia may go through a phase of eating excessively and may put on a great deal of weight, particularly if they are not active. This is a potential problem, and those caring for the person should reduce portion sizes accordingly.

- *Eating and drinking are activities!* We should always remember that we eat and drink for enjoyment as much as (or more than) nutritional reasons, and we should help people with dementia gain enjoyment from their meals. Make mealtimes pleasant occasions and opportunities for conversation and socialisation, and don't be afraid to eat out if that is something that the person used to enjoy.

As dementia progresses to the advanced phase, other issues may occur such as swallowing difficulties or the person may become unable to feed themselves. We will address these issues in Chapter 10.

## CHALLENGES WITH USING THE TOILET AND MANAGING CONTINENCE

People with dementia will find difficulties with using the toilet as embarrassing and distressing as this is for family members and friends. As dementia progresses, people may develop difficulties in passing urine or faeces, or both, and become incontinent as a result. Those caring for a person whose dementia has progressed will inevitably need to grasp the nettle of assisting the person with their continence needs, and how they do so will have a strong influence on the person's well-being and sense of dignity.

Broadly speaking, difficulties with using the toilet may result from three main causes, outlined below.

## Causes of continence problems
### Recognition and orientation
In early dementia, the person is aware of their need to go to the toilet and most of the time manages to use the toilet successfully. However, increasing memory, attention and executive function impairment may affect the person's ability to go to the toilet independently. A number of obstacles may present themselves:

- Difficulty with expressing a need to go to the toilet, or asking where the toilet is

- Being unable to find their way to the toilet

- Setting off for the toilet but then forgetting where they were going

- Leaving it too late to go to the toilet and/or to adjust their clothing in time

- Difficulty with recognising the toilet, due to visual-perceptual problems

- Successfully using the toilet, but then have difficulty in cleaning themselves and re-adjusting their clothing.

These challenges may result in the person having an 'accident', with consequent embarrassment and possible bad feelings.

### Physical health causes

The person's need to go to the toilet may be heightened by physical health issues such as urinary tract infections, stomach upsets, prostate problems in men, weakened bladder muscles in women who have had children, constipation, strokes, poor mobility or medications that increase urine output (diuretics). These can all lead to the person needing to go to the toilet more urgently than usual and less time to use the toilet successfully.

### Progression of dementia

In the later phases of dementia, the person's awareness of their need to go to the toilet diminishes and is eventually lost. When this happens, the person becomes *doubly incontinent*. We will consider this situation in Chapter 10.

'My wife started having problems with continence; she seemed to be frightened of going to the toilet and was only going about once a fortnight. She had also started having problems finding the toilet. On one occasion she got into a terrible state and I eventually persuaded her and got her in the toilet and left her in there, but when I went back the walls were covered, she was covered...it was awful.' (Family member)

## Helping a person with dementia meet their continence needs

This will challenge family members' and friends' qualities of tolerance and acceptance, but it is important that an open, accepting and non-blaming attitude is adopted if the person starts to have 'accidents'. Those caring for the person may need to take a proactive approach to helping the person with using the toilet. Principles for assisting the person meet their needs will depend on the person's particular difficulties, and may include the following:

- If the person has an accident, respond in an accepting and non-blaming way. Help the person clean themselves up.

- Ascertain the actual difficulties that the person has. The person may be able to tell you what they feel the problem is, but if not, observe them going to the toilet (embarrassing though that may be), which may offer clues.

- If there is a possible physical health cause (this may particularly be the case if the person suddenly starts having more accidents than usual), consult the person's GP.

- If the person is inclined to forget about going to the toilet, try tactfully reminding them. You could try saying, 'I'm dying for the loo, what about you?'

Individual solutions are likely to be needed for the person's specific difficulties. If they can't find their way to the toilet, signs may help. Try leaving the door open or show them the way. Contrasting colour toilet seats, towels and toilet paper will all help with recognition. If managing clothing is the problem, clothes that are easy to remove and put back on will help. In all cases an open, accepting but tactful and respectful manner on the part of family members and friends will help spare the person from embarrassment, and will maximise their ability to maintain independence in meeting their continence needs.

In some cases, continence pads may be a practical solution to avoiding the embarrassment and inconvenience of accidents. Elasticated pull-up pads are available that may be helpful for people who are starting to lose control over their bladder and bowels. These look and feel like normal underpants, are easy to use and people with dementia usually tolerate them well. We will discuss the use of pads further in Chapter 10.

'My husband couldn't remember how to use the zip on his trousers, so we chose tracksuit bottoms.' (Family member)

## CHALLENGES DUE TO SLEEP DISTURBANCES

Disturbances in sleeping patterns are common amongst people with dementia and can become more of an issue as dementia progresses. This can be especially difficult for those living with the person who may also have their sleep disturbed. For people with dementia with Lewy bodies or Parkinson's disease, sleep disturbance can be particularly prevalent, but all types of dementia can affect sleeping.

'Sleep is a big problem for me now. I have nightmares which I never used to have.' (Person with dementia)

### Causes of sleep disturbances

It is important to try and understand what may be causing the problem in order to decide which strategies might help. In the first instance, keeping a diary may be useful in establishing what the pattern is and what is happening to the person during the day. Factors that can contribute towards disturbed sleep include:

- Physical health problems such as urine infections or prostrate problems that may lead to an increased need to use the toilet

- Pain or discomfort, including arthritis and leg cramps

- Reduced need for sleep or sleeping too much during the day

- Depression, which can cause early morning wakening

- Environmental disturbances, for example poor lighting, noise or inappropriate temperature

- Nightmares or night terrors

- Restless leg syndrome or uncontrolled limb movements – these symptoms are commonly experienced by people with dementia with Lewy bodies or Parkinson's disease.

## Helping someone achieve a more settled sleep pattern

Whilst there may be no easy solution to sleep disturbances, it is essential that the possible causes are investigated so that those who are doing the caring can also get their much-needed sleep. Going without sleep must be one of the most difficult things to cope with for all concerned, and is likely to increase irritability for anyone. Some suggestions for achieving a more settled sleep pattern are offered here:

- Ask for a physical health check if there are any signs or symptoms of ill health that might be causing the person's sleep pattern to be disturbed.

- Try to establish a regular routine if possible, which includes exercise in the morning, and avoid difficult tasks that may cause distress in the late afternoon or early evening.

- Ensure adequate light and activity during the day, as this helps establish a good sleep pattern.

- Try to avoid long periods of sleep during the day.

- Avoid consumption of caffeine and alcohol in the evening.

- Consider whether medications are causing sleep problems – AChE inhibitor drugs can cause night-time stimulation and dream disturbance, so should be taken in the morning.

- Check the temperature of the bedroom is comfortable – not too hot or too cold.

- Use low-level or night lights to help the person find the bathroom and promote orientation.

- If the person is in an unfamiliar environment, try to put familiar things in sight such as photos or prized possessions.

- Play soft music as they go to sleep.

- Try using lavender oil in a diffuser, or put a few drops on the person's pillow.

If the person continues to have disturbed sleep or refuses to go to bed at a reasonable time, try to be flexible: let them sleep on the sofa or make sure the house is safe if they walk around in the night. It may be necessary for those who are caring to sleep in a separate bed or room if possible, to avoid both people having a disturbed night.

Sleep disturbances may be a stage the person with dementia goes through that will subside and settle over time. As dementia progresses further, people tend to sleep more. If problems persist, medical advice may be sought about night-time sedation, although this is generally not advised for people with dementia due to risk of increased confusion. A short-term trial of sleeping tablets may help with re-establishing a routine, but should be monitored carefully.

## CHALLENGES OF HOSPITAL ADMISSION

As the majority of people with dementia are older people and therefore more prone to physical illness, it follows that a person with dementia may, at some time, be admitted to a general hospital. As dementia itself may make the person more vulnerable to physical conditions, the numbers are high: in the UK, approximately 25 per cent of all general hospital beds at any time are occupied by people with dementia. In this section we consider the issues facing the person with dementia and their family and friends if the person is admitted to a general hospital (we don't discuss the care of people with dementia who are reaching the end of life in this section, as this is addressed in Chapter 11).

## What leads to people with dementia being admitted to hospital?

The most common reasons for admission to general hospital are:

- Fractured hip following a fall
- Urinary tract infection (UTI)
- Chest infection (including pneumonia)
- Stroke
- Generally failure to thrive, including loss of weight or self-neglect.

These conditions are common in older people, but people with dementia may be particularly likely to experience them. Infections and other conditions may lead to the person experiencing delirium (see Chapter 3), which may lead to a temporary rise in 'confusion', disorientation and memory difficulties – people with dementia are particularly prone to episodes of delirium when physically unwell.

The risk of the person developing these conditions may be reduced if the person is well looked after, well nourished and exercises regularly (but safely, to avoid falls). If the person does experience infections such as UTIs or pneumonia, these may be treatable in the person's home or care home setting. Some GPs refer people with dementia to hospital too readily, without properly considering community-based treatment and care.

## Issues for people with dementia in general hospitals

Avoiding hospital admission if possible is important as there is strong evidence that people with dementia do not fare well in general hospitals – people with dementia spend longer in hospital, recover less quickly and have higher mortality rates than people of similar ages and conditions who do not have dementia. A period in hospital may lead to the person entering residential care prematurely due to poor recovery. The person may lack awareness of the fact that they are ill and may well not cooperate with treatment. Furthermore, general hospitals are not good environments for people with dementia. Hospital wards are noisy, unfamiliar and confusing places that are rarely conducive to their needs. It can also be difficult for people with dementia to walk about safely in a hospital ward or find their way around. People with dementia may be unable to find their way to the toilet on a hospital ward or ask staff for help, leading to an increased frequency of accidents. It is small wonder that many people with dementia experience increased distress and anxiety, further compromising their recovery.

'I am worried that hospital admission will result in confusion, disorientation, anxiety, loss of any sort of control. I will need my family to advocate for me when I cannot do so myself.' (Person with dementia)

Another factor that can affect recovery in general hospitals is that staff can be unprepared for caring for people with dementia. Research has shown that many general nurses receive little education in their nurse training about caring for people with dementia. A particular issue is eating and drinking. General hospital staff can sometimes be unaware that the person's cognitive difficulties can compromise their ability to give themselves adequate nourishment, and sometimes don't offer appropriate assistance. Lack of understanding amongst staff of appropriate ways of interacting with people with dementia or responding to distressed behaviour can lead to excessive use of sedative medication, further compromising the person's physical health. Difficulties faced by staff in general hospitals include inadequate staffing levels and the fact that the focus of care is often 'fast-paced' and geared towards acute illness rather than long-term conditions such as dementia.

Improving general hospital care and preventing avoidable admissions is an important way to improve the experience for people with dementia and their families. Improving the understanding of staff, enhancing assessment and recognition of dementia, involving families in care, changing the environment and making care individualised are all important ways in which care can be improved. The National Dementia Action Alliance (NDAA) has produced a charter, including a summary of what families should expect (see the Resources section at the end of the book for further information).

## How can family members and friends help?

How family members and friends can help improve the experience of people with dementia in general hospitals in many ways matches their contribution if the person receives residential care, and we will discuss these principles in Chapter 9. Some approaches are listed below:

- Tell hospital staff about the person, their past life (so that staff have a better appreciation of them as individuals), their likes and dislikes, and any tips or strategies for assisting with aspects of care. Many hospitals have documents called *personal profiles*, such as 'This is me' (see the Resources section), that are used to record this information. These should be kept in an accessible place so that staff can see them, but families have an important role in reminding people to do this.

- Offer assistance with things such as eating and drinking or helping the person use the toilet, if appropriate.

- Spending time with the person and doing activities will help relieve boredom and distress. Many hospitals now invite family carers to stay with the person, including overnight, and have open visiting hours. This said, it might also be important for those who are the main carer to have a rest, so asking other family members and friends to help out with visiting is important.

Above all, people with dementia should be given the best opportunity to recover from physical illness, and family members and friends may sometimes need to be assertive with hospital staff to ensure that appropriate care standards are maintained.

## CHALLENGES OF VULNERABILITY AND ABUSE

Due to reduced or lack of mental capacity, people with dementia are particularly vulnerable to the risk of harm, as the ability to understand their situation, make decisions and look after themselves will all become significantly impaired as the condition progresses. We have discussed situations where the person may come to harm due to their own actions, but we must also be aware that people with dementia may be at risk of harm from others – including those who are in a caring relationship with the person, such as family members, friends and professional carers. In the UK, the Care Act (2014) has established a legal framework for safeguarding vulnerable adults, including people with dementia, from abuse and neglect, with clear responsibilities for local authorities and other bodies.

Types of abuse include the following:

- *Physical abuse:* We will all surely agree that if you hit, kick or slap a person with dementia, then you have abused that person. Furthermore, if you acted in this way towards an older person, the harm caused would be disproportionately great if the person was physically frail.

- *Psychological abuse:* Within this category are included threats of harm or abandonment, deprivation of contact, humiliation, blaming, controlling, intimidation, coercion, harassment and verbal abuse. Some of these have echoes of Tom Kitwood's categories of malignant social psychology, discussed earlier, in Chapter 6. People with dementia may be particularly affected, as they are less likely to be able to defend themselves or answer back.

- *Sexual abuse:* This includes rape and sexual assault, or sexual acts to which the vulnerable adult has not consented, or could not consent, or was pressured into consenting. We may feel that sexual abuse of older people in general and people with dementia in particular is unlikely to happen, but not many years ago it was also widely believed that sexual abuse of children rarely happened. The problem of obtaining consent when someone has limited capacity means that people whose dementia has progressed are at increased risk of sexual abuse.

- *Financial or material abuse:* This includes theft, fraud, exploitation, pressure in connection with wills, property or inheritance, or financial transactions, or the misuse or misappropriation of property, possessions or benefits. People with dementia are especially vulnerable to financial abuse, particularly if they have built up savings. Research suggests that financial exploitation of older people by their own families is depressingly common. Anyone who has attempted to acquire power of attorney for a person with dementia will know how complex the application process is, largely to try to safeguard the person against exploitation. People outside the family may exploit people with dementia financially, as the person's reduced capacity for decision-making may cause them to make unwise financial arrangements. Unscrupulous individuals may 'befriend' the person with the intention of getting money from them, and we are also familiar with news reports of tradespeople or doorstep salespeople charging extortionate fees for services that the person does not need.

- *Neglect and acts of omission:* This includes ignoring medical or physical care needs, failure to provide access to appropriate health or social care services, and the withholding of the necessities of life, such as medication, adequate nutrition or heating. We have discussed above how people with dementia come to rely on others to meet their daily living needs and the complexities that may arise in helping people with dementia meet those needs. Again, failure by those caring for a person with dementia to fulfil their caring responsibilities is sadly not uncommon.

- *Discriminatory abuse:* This is perhaps an unexpected category, but it is nevertheless an important one when considering people with dementia. It embraces comments or actions that are racist or sexist, based on a person's disability, and other forms of harassment, slurs or similar treatment. People with dementia may be on the receiving end of racial or sexual slurs, as may the rest of us, and as stated above, may lack the ability to defend themselves. In addition, they may also experience discrimination due to having dementia. We have observed that the public's view of dementia, reflected in the media, is often a negative one, and people with dementia are sometimes described in pejorative terms – 'gaga', 'gone back to childhood', etc. We have also heard of people with dementia who have been refused access to pubs and restaurants on account of their condition.

## What can family members and friends do if they suspect that a person with dementia is being abused?

This is a difficult question to answer, and it may depend on the nature of the suspicions and whether the alleged abuse is being carried out by a family member or carer or by professional care staff (we will touch on abuse and neglect in care homes in Chapter 9). The nature of dementia means that the person is less likely to be able to complain that they are being abused, or if they do so, they may not be believed. It is also possible that they may not be aware that abuse is taking place. Also, families are complicated entities, and interfering with long-standing relationships, even if those relationships appear to be dysfunctional, may not necessarily be in the person's best interests. At the same time, you should not stand back and let a person with dementia suffer abuse or neglect – it is not unknown for older people to die as a result. Discussions within the family may help, or concerned individuals could contact their local authority social services department. Charities exist to offer confidential advice (for example, Action on Elder Abuse), and if it is felt that the situation is serious, then the police should be contacted. Abusing or neglecting a vulnerable adult is a criminal offence.

# CHAPTER 9

# Considering Residential Care for People with Dementia

## PERCEPTIONS OF RESIDENTIAL CARE

Care homes sadly often receive negative press coverage, and we may hold significant concerns about whether residential care is right for the person we care for, as stories of drab, unstimulating, neglectful and sometimes downright abusive care homes crop up from time to time. However, many care homes today are bright, welcoming, well-run establishments, with staff who are skilled in dementia care and who have residents' best interests at heart. For some people with dementia, going to live in a care home can be a positive experience that enhances their well-being and quality of life – and that also benefits their families and friends.

This is not to say that all people who reach a certain point in their dementia should, as a matter of course, go to live in a care home. As described in Chapter 4, there are increasingly varied sources of support available in 'the community', such as extra care, retirement or dementia villages where people may live, even as their dementia progresses. Others may be able to access a high level of support at home. However, for some people these options may not be possible due a number of factors, including the extent of their needs, the support that is available and their finances. This is when a care home is usually considered, although the principle of doing what is in the person's best interests should always be used to inform decisions.

The decision to look for a care home is a complex and often difficult one, and every family will need to make that decision through close consideration of individual circumstances. This can be particularly difficult for younger people with dementia, as care homes are rarely available to meet the specific needs of this group.

Not all care homes are alike. The decision about which care home to choose can be as hard as the decision to consider a care home in the first place and financial considerations can loom large. Families may need to argue their case quite strongly with social workers when asking for a care home they feel best meets the needs of the person.

In this section we consider some of the many factors that families must take into account in making these decisions. We also consider how family and friends can maintain relationships with the person once they are living in a care home.

## WHAT IS RESIDENTIAL CARE?

The term *care home* is used to cover any formal setting where people live and are looked after by paid staff. Care homes are usually categorised either as *residential* or *nursing* homes, the difference being the extent of nursing needs that can be provided for. Some care homes are specifically approved for people with dementia, although they are often supported well in other care home settings. Care homes are largely owned and managed by private companies rather than by the public sector. Companies vary greatly in size, from large national concerns that own hundreds of homes to independent providers that may own just one or two. Payment arrangements for people living in care homes can be complex, but often the person themselves (or their family on their behalf) must pay some or all of the costs, depending on their savings and assets.

Research shows that the majority of older people want to live in their own homes, or with their families, rather than in care homes, and surveys of family carers indicate that this is what they would prefer as well. It is understandable that if possible people would want to live in surroundings that are private and familiar, and with their families rather than with strangers.

> 'My family know I don't want to go into residential care or for them to look after me. I've been on my own for most of my life, so to suddenly be surrounded by other people and noises would be quite disturbing, I imagine.' (Person with dementia)

The negative image of care homes also undoubtedly contributes to the preference for staying at home. In addition, care homes are expensive, both for individuals and for governments that must fund those who cannot pay for themselves. In the UK only around one-third of people with dementia live in care homes, despite sometimes having extensive care needs.

## THE DECISION

There are many families and friends who continue to care for people with dementia at home throughout the progression of the person's condition, and we will discuss some of the principles of caring for people with advanced dementia in the next chapter. However, in some situations a care home may be the best place for the person to live, and family and friends should not feel guilty about taking that step. Indeed, some people may have made an active decision to go into a care home if their needs become too great for the family to cope with. Living in a care home will not necessarily lead to the person experiencing a poorer quality of life and sense of well-being, and good care homes can be pleasant, stimulating and enjoyable places. In short, a move to a care home may be the best thing for the person and for their family and friends.

> 'My husband has made the decision to go into care later on, regardless of how we the family felt. He has taken the decision,

> and therefore lifted any quandary or guilt from our shoulders.' (Family member)

> 'I was encouraged by the social worker to start having a look at nursing homes just to see what was out there; this was very traumatic but I went to have a look at a few places; on reflection it helped prepare me.' (Family member)

In order for this outcome to be achieved, family and friends must think through the issues and plan the move carefully. Sometimes this is not possible if the move comes about as a result of a crisis situation, such as a sudden deterioration in the person's health or the health of their main carer. In most cases, however, a move to a care home will have been considered more or less openly for some time.

## Involving the person with dementia in the decision

As discussed in Chapter 5, it is helpful to have discussed and recorded the person's preferences for future care in an 'advance statement' document whilst they are still able to clearly express their views.

> 'The type of care home that I'd want would be one where I am involved in activities as much as possible and treated with love and care.' (Person with dementia)

Not everyone will have expressed their preference about future care before the condition has progressed, making the decision more difficult. The concern may be that the person will either not understand what is being suggested to them or will immediately say 'no', through not wanting to leave their home or not recognising the risks of staying in their own home if their support needs cannot be met.

It is also not uncommon for people to say they would not want to become a 'burden' to their families. The person might have given permission to family and friends to seek residential care for them in certain circumstances, and may express preferences about where they would like to live.

Even if the person's dementia has progressed, we should not assume that the decision cannot be discussed with them. They may retain enough awareness to understand the implications of what is being proposed and may not necessarily disagree, recognising at some level that such a move may be for the best. The transition to a care home may be easier if the person has been prepared as far as possible for the move. Sometimes, however, the decision has to be taken by family and friends in the person's best interests and without their consent or even their awareness.

> 'We're past the point where grandma can participate in any decisions. I know she wants to stay at home but...' (Family member)

## Making the decision

The decision-making process will be different for each family and will be easier for some than others. Sometimes the decision will, in effect, be taken out of their hands, if the person's main carer (who may well be an elderly spouse or partner) becomes ill or even dies and no one else is able to take on the caring role. In such cases an emergency admission to hospital is often the first step to the person's move to a care home, although this is not desirable.

For others, the decision is far from easy, and the nature of the relationship is likely to be an important factor. A husband or wife may not want to be parted from their life partner, or an adult child may feel guilty about giving up caring for their parent. Other family members may exert subtle pressure on the main carer's sense of duty, and cultural factors may come into play as well, particularly amongst some minority ethnic groups. The person themselves may give out the message that they want to stay at home, thereby adding to the carer's sense of responsibility. Family members, rightly or wrongly, may feel that they are condemning the person to a life of unhappiness or worse if they enter a care home. They may feel that nurses and paid carers cannot possibly know the person as well as them and will not be able to care as effectively and sensitively.

'I am worried about lack of care in the care home. I am sure I will be that obstructive wife causing problems for the staff but in support of my husband, but then I will have to leave him alone afterwards. That is a concern. Will I be brave enough, and will they behave differently when I am not there?' (Family member)

'Dementia, by its nature, presents a series of losses over time. The biggest loss was actually when my husband went in the care home. For the first time we were living apart, it felt like a death, but a line hadn't been drawn under it and you feel very bereaved.' (Family member)

On the other hand, caring for a person with dementia can be difficult and sometimes stressful and exhausting. As we saw in Chapter 8, the person's manner and behaviour may cause difficulties. Helping the person with activities of daily living such as dressing, nutrition and keeping clean can be tiring. Sometimes the person's actions may put themselves or others at risk, and maintaining vigilance can be exhausting for carers. It may be particularly difficult and distressing for family and friends if the person becomes incontinent, and this, for some, can be the 'straw that breaks the camel's back'.

Carers must also cope with the emotional aspects of caring – seeing a person they have known and loved for years changing in front of them and sometimes not appreciating what is being done for them. They may well also have to manage changes in other relationships. Family tensions can be exacerbated by caring, and friendships can sometimes be broken when friends stop visiting. Adult children may have given up work in order to care, or will have no time for their own hobbies or interests. It is unsurprising that research has shown that carers of people with dementia report more stress (physical, emotional and financial) than those in other caring roles, and have greater rates of physical and mental health problems than those of similar ages and backgrounds who do not have a caring role.

For some, however, the benefits of maintaining the caring role outweigh the drawbacks. Their emotional ties to the person with dementia may be strong enough for them to cope or their support network may sustain them. Some people do not regard the caring role as especially difficult at all – they get a sense of satisfaction and purpose from caring, and continue to look after the person at home long after the person would qualify for a care home. For many others, however, the point is reached when the stress becomes too great, or the sheer practicalities of caring too difficult, even with professional help. The decision is made, ideally with the contribution and support of other family members and friends and in conjunction with advice from professionals such as social workers or the person's GP, but sometimes alone.

'I'd like my husband to stay at home for as long as possible but I'm not going to be a martyr about it, if it came to the point that he needed more care than I can give him.' (Family member)

'My sisters and I could see that dad was getting tired but he would never say it was getting too much. We could see he was struggling, so we got the social worker to come to the house for a meeting with us and she put it to dad about mum going into permanent residential care. He got upset and started to cry and said he didn't want to feel he'd given up on her.' (Family member)

## CHOOSING A CARE HOME

Family and friends, as well as the person themselves wherever possible, should have a measure of choice regarding where the person with dementia goes to live. Unfortunately this is not always the case, and families may need to negotiate carefully with the local authority. A care needs assessment should be carried out to determine the level of support the person needs, including residential, nursing and/or dementia-specific care. Highlighting the specific needs of the person and what is in their best interests is important, including locality so that family members and friends can visit regularly. Ultimately, though, availability and cost will play a significant part.

The factors involved in making the choice will differ, with some families placing greater weight on particular aspects than others. In this section we attempt to guide families and friends through the issues of selecting a care home, with or on behalf of a person with dementia.

## CARE HOME FEES

One of the first considerations will undoubtedly be finance, as the cost of residential care is not cheap. The costs also vary significantly between different care home providers and areas, and will understandably be an influencing factor on the decision. The first step will include a financial assessment by the local council about how much you need to contribute towards care home fees. The rules about how much funding is available from either social services or the NHS are complex and are a subject of much debate and controversy. Generally, the more money a person has in savings, the less financial support they will receive. This includes the value of someone's home if owned and if leaving the property vacant. If a family member is still living there, the value would generally not be included if that person is under 18, over 60 or is disabled. It is possible that selling someone's home can be deferred, but how this is managed may vary according to different local councils. Strict rules are, however, applied about not passing on a house or savings to others in order to avoid care home fees, which is referred to as deliberate *deprivation of assets*.

There is a requirement, however, that the person's assets are not reduced to below a certain amount, with numerous lobbies suggesting putting a cap on how much someone should pay.

If the person does not own their own home and has less than the specified amount of savings, funding should be made available, although top-up fees may be required if the care home fees are over and above what is offered. Additionally, if someone requires full nursing care, an assessment should be carried out to access some NHS funding. Sometimes families decide to contribute towards care home fees if they want a specific care home that is more expensive than the local authority will fund. Whilst this is understandable if a family can afford to do so, careful consideration is needed about how long top-up fees may be required.

In summary, this is a complex issue and the rules are often changing, so we would strongly advise readers to seek advice and refer to useful websites such as that of Age UK that provide the most up-to-date guidance (see the Resources section at the end of the book).

## HOW TO FIND OUT ABOUT CARE HOMES

There are a large number of care homes in the UK. Local authorities keep lists, or information may be found in the local library or on the internet.[1] Basic information that families and friends need includes:

- The owning company – is it a large or small concern?

- Will the home meet the person's needs? What level of nursing care does it provide, and does it have a specialised dementia care facility?

- What are the fees? Is the home affordable?

- Is it a large home divided into several units or a small single-unit facility?

- How many beds does the home have?

---

1   See the Resources section at the end of the book for further information.

- Where is the home situated? Is it easy for family and friends to visit?

- Does the home have grounds and gardens?

- Does the home state that activities are provided?

This kind of basic information will be available from a home's website or brochure but says nothing about the quality of the home and the care it offers. Families and friends must use other sources of information regarding these aspects. Social workers or other professionals may be unable to make specific recommendations, so families and friends must find out in other ways:

- *Personal recommendation:* In many aspects of life, recommendations from trusted people are often the best way of ascertaining the quality of services, and care homes are no different. It is worth asking around to find someone who can offer advice from their own experience.

- *Official reports:* In England and Wales the Care Quality Commission (CQC) inspects and approves care homes, and their reports are available on the internet. In Scotland the equivalent body is the Care Inspectorate, and in Northern Ireland, the Regulation and Quality Improvement Authority. Whilst these reports may offer some important information, they only give impressions based on sometimes brief inspection visits, and may not get below the surface of a home.

- *Reviews on the internet:* carehome.co.uk includes an increasing number of reviews written by family members and friends of residents of individual homes, and rates homes on a 1–10 scale based on those reviews. These should not be taken too literally, but may be helpful, along with other sources of information.

- *Visiting the home and talking to staff:* Just as we would not buy a house without viewing it, we should not decide on a place for a person with dementia to live without visiting it and looking around. We recommend visiting several homes to build up an impression of what is available and to make comparisons. No care home is perfect, and there may be difficulties lurking under the surface, but much can be ascertained from a carefully planned and conducted visit.

## WHAT SHOULD BE EXPECTED OF A CARE HOME?

Family members and friends will get the best out of a visit to a care home by talking to staff and looking around to observe the environment and the people – staff and residents. The fundamental questions to try to answer are straightforward:

* Will the person be known, understood and treated as an individual? Will the staff have an attitude of respect and of wanting the best for their residents? Will they know their residents, not just in the present, but in the context of their past lives? Will the care they give be adapted to the needs of each individual? What is being looked for is evidence of what the psychologist Tom Kitwood and others term 'person-centred care'.

* Will the person with dementia be looked after well? A baseline standard is that residents should be clean, well dressed and properly nourished with food and fluids. However, this must go hand-in-hand with other aspects of care: psychological, social and spiritual. There must be evidence that the home's staff are proactive in promoting these aspects as well as providing a good standard of physical care.

* Will the person have a good quality of life? As we have maintained throughout this book, this should embrace opportunities for interaction with others and meaningful activity. It should also include the opportunity to

experience different environments, including access to the open air.

- Will the person experience well-being? Whilst well-being cannot be guaranteed for any of us all the time, the sense of well-being for a person with dementia will be enhanced and maintained if the factors set out above are in place, and if the care home staff take proper steps to assist the person if they are distressed.

- Will families and friends be similarly respected? Family members and friends will have their own needs for information and support once a person goes to live in a care home, and may also have a lot to offer staff in terms of understanding the person and advice regarding aspects of care. Many will still want to be involved in the care of the person, and a good care home will embrace the principles of 'relationship-based care' – regarding family members and friends as partners in caring for residents.

In seeking to achieve these aims, care home staff must show that they do *not* display what Tom Kitwood terms a 'standard paradigm' approach to people with dementia. Evidence of this includes:

- Staff displaying negative attitudes towards residents or a lack of sensitivity towards their needs – sometimes this includes staff cutting corners or organising their working day to suit themselves rather than residents.

- Staff who concern themselves with physical or daily living-based care only, ignoring the social, psychological or spiritual sides of care; along with this goes lack of knowledge of residents as individuals.

- Care regimes that are 'one size fits all' rather than being individualised, with an over-reliance on routines and a lack of flexibility.

- The use of sedating medication (or even physical restraints) as a response to distressed behaviour, rather than staff trying to understand that behaviour and finding creative ways of meeting the person's underlying needs.

- Family members and friends being ignored, patronised or excluded, and questions or complaints not taken seriously.

No care home is perfect and resources may be limited in some care homes, which can lead to compromises in the delivery of care. However, the ideals of person-centred care are no more than any of us would want or expect, and so evidence should be present that the balance of care in a home is skewed much more towards 'person-centred' care rather than the 'standard paradigm'.

## VISITING A CARE HOME: A CHECKLIST OF WHAT TO LOOK FOR

When visiting a care home, try to make a judgement about the quality of care the home provides. Whilst it is very difficult to do this precisely, by taking note of some important aspects as listed below, family and friends can gain as clear an idea as possible.

### Talk to the manager

Much research has shown that the manager of any kind of care facility, whether it is a hospital ward or a care home, is crucial for setting the tone of that facility and marking out the quality standards expected of staff:

- Make sure you talk to the home manager, and if the home has a number of separate units, the manager of the unit where the person would live.

- Ask them about their philosophy of care and what they want for their residents. Look for key words in their answer such as person-centred care, quality of life and well-being.

- Ask them how they ensure that their staff fulfil that philosophy – a good manager will spend time on the 'shop floor' working directly with staff and residents.

- If the manager shows you around, look for how they talk to staff and residents whilst they do so: can you see evidence of mutual respect?

If the manager is 'too busy' to see you, don't bother visiting.

## Find out about the staff

- Ask about the staff – numbers, turnover, qualifications, experience and specific training in dementia care.

- Ask to be introduced to some staff members. Do they seem happy in their job?

- As you go around, look at what the staff are doing. Are they interacting with the residents or are they huddled together in the staff office?

- What is the quality of the interaction? Is it respectful, caring and person-centred?

## Observe residents' well-being

It is useful as you go around to take note of what residents are doing and how contented they appear:

- Are the residents clean and presentable, and do they appear to be well nourished?

- Do they appear to be distressed? If so, how are they responded to?

- Are they alert and active? If a high proportion of residents are asleep during the day, this may suggest an unstimulating environment or over-use of sedative medication.

• If residents have advanced dementia and physical frailty (see Chapter 10), are they comfortable?

• Is it apparent staff have taken steps to get to know residents as people and to maintain their sense of individuality?

• Ask how staff find out about residents' previous lives and see if residents have personal belongings and things important to their identity, such as family photographs or life story profiles.

## Look for evidence of activities

Ask about the provision of social and recreational activities, and look for evidence that they are actually taking place. Most good homes will employ an activity coordinator, but ideally all staff should be involved in activities:

• Are residents taking part in activities during your visit, or is it apparent that activities actually take place?

• Is it evident that residents have the opportunity to exercise outdoors?

## What is the physical environment like?

The home's design and environment is important in promoting well-being in people with dementia:

• Are the lights bright but not glaring?

• Have attempts been made to help residents maintain orientation, such as clear signs to toilets and bedrooms?

• Is extraneous noise minimised?

• Is there space where residents can walk about safely?

- Are there communal areas but also enough space that residents don't feel crowded out by each other?

- Is the decor and furniture homely and in good condition? Are residents' rooms comfortable and personalised?

- Are there pictures on the walls, and are they likely to be of interest to residents?

- Can you see evidence of objects that support activity such as games, books, music or occupational tools?

## Attitude towards families and friends

A good home will welcome families and friends and will not restrict their visiting. Furthermore, a good home will encourage families to participate in care giving and will show concern for their needs.

- Ask the manager if this is the case.

- If possible, ask to speak to the relatives of residents, if any happen to be visiting.

## Judge the home's 'feel'

Sometimes it is possible to pick up the ambience of a home as soon as you walk through the front door. Some 'feel' good and others don't. Little things may come together to create a positive or negative 'feel'.

- Smell is an obvious indicator. With doubly incontinent residents, some smell of urine or faeces may be inevitable, but if that smell hits you strongly as soon as you walk in, that may be a sign that staff have been leaving residents unattended for too long.

- Noise is another sign – is there a lot of shouting out by residents (or even by staff)? A subtle trick is to listen to what station the radio is tuned to – if it is blaring out pop music, it is likely that young care staff have tuned it to a channel that they want to listen to rather than one that is appropriate for the residents.

- Does the home appear to be a lively place? Are there plants and pets and even dolls and games?

- How welcoming or otherwise are staff when they see you? Do they have good 'front of house' skills? Does it feel genuine?

At the end of the day, a good care home will be like a good hotel – welcoming, relaxing and efficient, with a range of activities and choice, and evidence that the staff value their residents and want the best for them.

'One of the things I would look at is the turnover of staff – if it is low and the staff are happy to remain, something must be right.' (Family member)

## MAKING THE TRANSITION

The transition from living at home to living in a care home may well not be easy for either the person with dementia or their family. Proper preparation will help to make the transition as smooth as possible.

As discussed above, involving the person in the decision to enter residential care can be awkward. Some families do not ask or tell the person with dementia of their intention to seek a care home place, thinking that the person will either not understand or will resist the idea. Whilst this approach may be understandable, it can make the transition more difficult. Broaching the subject may, however, be problematic if the person's cognitive difficulties are such that they cannot understand the concept of a care home. It is a good idea for the person themselves to visit the homes on the family's shortlist along with the family carer (this should be after the family has made a first exploratory visit), to see if they appear to like and feel settled in each home.

> 'In an ideal scenario, you would know what to expect. It'd be good to have an experience of a care home, to try it out; for it to be positive and for my wife to be supported.' (Person with dementia)

How this is introduced to the person will depend on circumstances; some will go along with the family willingly, whilst others may be suspicious of where they are going. If someone is unable to recognise that they need the support of a care home, they may be unwilling to go along with the decision. In these situations, the principles of truth telling, as outlined in Chapter 6, may be helpful, in that you should start by sensitively telling the truth, but if it causes distress, try different approaches along the continuum, using 'untruths' if required.

> 'I spoke to my wife about it and I told her that I had spoken to the doctor and that she needed to go into a clinic; she was happy with this.' (Family member)

Sooner or later the choice of home will be made and arrangements for the move put into place. Sometimes the person will go for a trial period, to see if they settle into the home and it meets their needs; in other cases a clean transition is made. Family and friends can ease the transition through keeping the person as aware of events as possible, by trying not to appear distressed themselves and by working with the home's staff to help the person settle in. Coordinating the move with staff is important. The person should be expected and welcomed by the home's staff, shown around and helped with their belongings. Familiar clothes and objects will help relieve the person's anxieties and suspicions, and family members can help the person unpack and put things away in their room (again, some people with dementia may believe they are staying at a hotel and it may be helpful for them to do so). When saying goodbye, again, maintain a calm and reassuring manner, and tell the person you will be back to see them soon.

'I took my wife into her room; the carers came in and they were lovely and they said to me that the best thing was that I should go. She looked a little bit concerned but was okay.' (Family member)

## STAYING INVOLVED

When a person with dementia goes to live in a care home, it does not mean that family members and friends have no further role to play, although sadly a minority will either visit infrequently or stop having any contact with the person. For the majority, however, moving to a care home simply begins a new phase. Family carers will have mixed feelings. Some may feel a measure of relief that some of their caring responsibilities have been lifted and they have more freedom for other aspects of their lives.

'When my mum went into a home it allowed me to be a daughter again, and it improved our relationship.' (Family member)

Others will feel a sense of loss, especially if the person with dementia is their spouse or partner, and may well also experience ongoing feelings of guilt at instigating the move, particularly if the person does not appear to be settled in their new home. The majority of family members and friends want to stay involved with the person's care, and a good care home will help them do so.

'I say to people that I am still a carer; just because I am not providing for my wife 24 hours a day doesn't mean that I don't care. I still make key decisions.' (Family member)

## Helping the transition

One way that family and friends can contribute to the person's care is by giving the care home staff information and advice about the person with dementia in order to help them get to know the person better and care for them more effectively. It is important that a person with dementia is understood in the context of the whole of their life, so that staff can appreciate and respect the person as an individual, and understand their actions and manner in relation to their biography. Many care homes compile fairly comprehensive life histories of new residents (see Chapter 5), and family members and friends are clearly the main sources of information for these exercises.

Good care home staff are also open to ideas from family and friends regarding aspects of caring for the person, and will welcome hints and strategies that family members can pass on based on their own experience of caring for the person. As we've also suggested, bringing in personal belongings, mementos and photographs (and also perhaps recordings of favourite music that staff can play to the person) will help the person settle and maintain their sense of identity.

## Visiting

Clearly the main way that family members and friends can stay involved is by visiting the person. Many people with dementia will continue to recognise their loved ones, even if they have little awareness of other aspects of their surroundings, and will 'light up' when familiar people arrive. Even if the person's condition has progressed so much that they no longer appear to know even those closest to them, visits will enhance the person's well-being (see Chapter 10). There are no hard and fast rules about how frequent visits should be – a few family members may visit every day – but all visits are valuable.

'The staff made a fuss of my dad as he visited mum every day; they'd make him his lunch and they were always very welcoming to him.' (Family member)

'My wife seemed to accept where she was and we visited every day; she has never asked how long she would be in for or ever asked to come home.' (Family member)

Visits can provide extra opportunities for activity as well as conversation, and if the person's language ability is impaired, then spending the time carrying out an activity may be more fruitful (see Chapter 7 for ideas). Good care homes will encourage families and friends to take residents out if possible, and will enable them to get involved in activities within the home.

Family members and friends can also assist with daily living activities. Homes should allow visitors to stay during mealtimes, and some family members enjoy helping the person eat their meals. Many people with dementia like to dress up and look their best, and again, visitors can sometimes assist in this area.

'If, when I visit, my wife's not good, I go away feeling terrible, but when she's happy I feel okay – I have spoken to other carers who say they feel the same.' (Family member)

## ISSUES WITH RESIDENTIAL CARE

We hope we have painted a positive picture of care homes in this chapter. There are many care homes with skilled, committed and empathic staff, and many people with dementia live lives in homes that are of good quality and promote well-being. Issues can arise, however, and we outline some of the more common ones here.

'It must go through everyone's mind about care homes – will I like it? Will I be looked after?' (Person with dementia)

### When the person does not settle

Good practice by care home staff in cooperation with family and friends will maximise the chances of the person with dementia settling into their new home. Sometimes, however, this does not happen. The person may appear to be distressed and agitated and may make frequent attempts to leave the home. Some may react aggressively to staff, particularly if staff do not approach the person in a sensitive way. In extreme circumstances the care home manager will decide that the person cannot stay at the home, and in most cases this is their prerogative.

This situation should be avoided by careful selection of a home, including family members being honest with the staff about the person's manner and actions and a well-managed transition period. Clearly a move to another home (sometimes preceded by an emergency hospital admission) is highly disruptive for the person, who may become even more unsettled following subsequent moves, but it should be acknowledged that this will occasionally occur.

In most cases the person will eventually settle, and family and friends can aid this process through working with the staff to come up with an individualised care plan for the person. Sometimes this may involve family and friends visiting more frequently, or it may involve less frequent visits if all agree that this is in the person's best interests.

## Deprivation of Liberty Safeguards (DoLS) or Liberty Protection Safeguards (LPS)

By the time a person with dementia enters a care home, they will often lack capacity related to major decisions (see Chapter 5). Staff may need to make significant care decisions such as preventing the person from leaving the home if it is unsafe for them to do so, or giving them personal care without their permission if their health is at risk.

In England and Wales a legal framework has been developed to allow care homes (and hospitals) to 'deprive the person of their liberty' in the legal sense. At the moment this is called 'Deprivation of Liberty Safeguards' (DoLS), but current proposals in government are suggesting amendments to change this to 'Liberty Protection Safeguards' (LPS). The principle in both is that an assessment is carried out to determine whether any restrictions being placed on the person, such as preventing the person from going outside, or the person being 'held' in order to provide care, are in the person's best interests, are proportionate and should be authorised or not. To determine this, the responsible body (under DoLS this is the local authority, but under LPS this may change) must consult with the person and others, to understand what the person's wishes and feelings about the arrangements are. A decision should be made about what is in the best interests of the person.

If anyone disagrees with the care arrangements or no one is available to represent the person who lacks capacity, an independent mental capacity professional should make an assessment. All decisions should be reviewed on a regular basis, which may be every one or three years (depending on the outcome of the current review of legislation). If there is any concern that someone's liberty or freedom is being restricted without proper authority, or that the person is at risk of abuse, family and friends should always seek advice from the local authority about possible safeguarding issues, as described in Chapter 8.

## Younger people with dementia in care homes

We discussed the specific issues related to younger people with dementia in Chapter 1. A proportion of those under the age of 65 who have dementia will require residential care. This can create problems as the numbers of such people in a given geographical area are likely to be very small and specialist residential care facilities are unlikely to be available. This means that younger people must often go to live in care homes that normally cater for older adults. This can be awkward for the person, who must live with people considerably older than themselves. It can also create challenges for staff as the person may be physically fitter and more active than other residents, may not appreciate the same activities as older residents, and may have particular care needs if they have a rarer form of dementia. Choice of home becomes particularly important in such cases, and family and friends may have a particular role to play in advising staff and supporting the person.

## Black, Asian and minority ethnic (BAME) groups and care homes

Research shows that minority ethnic groups are under-represented in care homes for people with dementia, implying that many families from these groups are caring for people in the later stage of dementia at home. As discussed in Chapter 1, there are likely to be a number of reasons for this. To recap, some ethnic groups have strong cultural values regarding looking after older family members within the family. Second, there may be stigma in some ethnic groups regarding dementia, and some families may feel ashamed if a member goes to live in a care home. Finally, and probably most importantly, minority ethnic families may feel that care homes that cater largely for the majority population may not offer culturally sensitive care to minorities. Suitable arrangements may not be made for food preferences, personal care, language issues and religious observance. There are no easy answers to this concern. Numbers of older people with dementia from minority ethnic groups are currently small, and there are few care homes that cater specifically for particular ethnic or religious groups. As in other aspects of their lives, those from minority ethnic groups who have dementia may face a harder battle to get their needs met in a society very different to their own.

## Lesbian, gay, bisexual and transgender (LGBT+) people with dementia and care homes

As mentioned in Chapter 1, the issues of care and support for LGBT+ people with dementia are the same as for others, but factors in their situation may create challenges if the person enters residential care. Some LGBT+ people may have become estranged from their families and enter residential care due to lack of support in the community. If the person has been living with and supported by a same-sex partner, that person will want to continue to visit and support the person. In theory there should not be an issue with this; the principles of relationship-based care should apply in all cases, and the person's partner should be welcomed by care home staff just as other family members and friends would be. In practice, attitudes can sometimes create barriers. Some care home staff may express negative attitudes towards LGBT+ people. Also, some couples may be reluctant to 'come out' to care home staff, either because they have always kept the nature of their relationship to themselves or through fear of possible negative reactions. Partnership with care home staff will be enhanced by a clear, shared understanding of the nature of the relationship between a resident and the person who regularly visits and provides support. Sometimes an open discussion with the home manager at the point of choosing a care home can facilitate that understanding, to the benefit of all concerned.

## Behaviour that care home staff find challenging

Just as family members and friends may find some aspects of the person's behaviour challenging, so do care home staff. If the person appears to be distressed or agitated, if they become aggressive, or if they persist in wanting to get away from the home, staff can feel as stressed as family members. The strategies that staff can use to respond to such behaviour are the same as those set out in Chapter 8, and should embrace an individualised approach based on knowing the person and their life history. Family members and friends can obviously contribute by telling staff about the person's life, and suggesting strategies that they have used in the past. Understanding the person's routines can help in adapting care: did they used to get up early for work, did they do night shifts or did they regularly pick children up from school at a certain time? Also knowing about previous roles and activities can help staff to understand behaviour – did they like to be outdoors, were they in positions of authority in their work, did they do manual labour?

Other difficulties can arise from the fact that the person is now living in a communal environment. Arguments may occur between residents if they lack sufficient space or are not supported adequately by staff. An issue that can sometimes arise is that of sexual relationships developing between residents. People with dementia can sometimes demonstrate sexual behaviour towards others without being aware of the implications. This can be challenging and needs to be responded to very carefully and sensitively. The onset of old age or a cognitive impairment does not take away the need for affection, intimacy or relationships, and care homes should have approaches that recognise this but also protect residents as potentially vulnerable.

Research suggests that some care home staff may resort to sedating medication as their main response to behaviour they find difficult, rather than looking for more person-centred solutions. This is despite the considerable drawbacks of such medication, discussed in Chapter 8. Family members and friends should ask the manager of a home at the initial visit how they respond to distressed or agitated behaviour, and what their attitude and approach is to the use of sedating medication.

## Concerns about standards of care

Family members and friends visiting the person may be critical of aspects of the care the person is receiving. Broadly speaking, such criticisms can arise for three main reasons, outlined below.

### Family members and friends believing that care is not up to their own standards

Many family carers provide a very high standard of care, particularly in terms of helping the person keep stimulated, clean, nourished and well presented. They may feel that the care home staff are not keeping up the standards they want or would provide themselves. They may feel that the person is dressed untidily, is not clean, or notice the person is losing weight. It is perhaps inevitable that hard-pressed care staff, who have to provide for many residents, may not be able to do things as well as a family member devoting their whole time to one person. At the same time, it is possible that standards are not as they should be at the home. This could be due to staff shortages, poorly trained staff or an ethos of cutting corners. A good relationship with the home or unit manager will help family and friends understand the home and its circumstances and make them feel that they can speak up if they sense that standards are slipping. Dialogue with the manager may also lead to family members assisting as appropriate with caring activities, such as supervising mealtimes.

### Differences of opinion regarding the most appropriate care

Sometimes the issue family members and friends have is not that the home is giving poor care, but that aspects of care are not as they would want it, or in their view, not what the person with dementia would want if they could express a choice. Perhaps the person's hair has been done differently, or they are eating (and apparently enjoying) food they would not normally eat, or taking part in activities they would not normally consider. Maybe the staff are responding to aspects of the person's behaviour in ways that family members do not regard as appropriate. In some cases family members and friends need to act as advocates for the person and inform staff of the person's preferences, for example if a life-long vegetarian is eating meat or the person is doing things that are against their long-held religious principles. In other cases it may be more appropriate to take a more open-minded and tolerant view. One situation that might arise is the care home staff using toys or dolls as a means of promoting activity (see Chapter 7). Family members may feel uncomfortable that their relative is playing with children's toys, but such activities may be appropriate for the person's abilities and may well enhance their well-being. Discussion with staff about the rationale for certain activities may help relieve family members' reservations about some aspects of dementia care that might appear inappropriate but that actually reflect good practice.

### Concerns about abusive, neglectful or exploitative practices

As discussed in Chapter 8, people with dementia are vulnerable to abuse, neglect and exploitation, and care home staff may, in rare cases, carry out such acts. If family members or friends suspect (or witness) that a member of staff is in some way abusing any resident, they should tell the manager at once, and if no action appears to be taken, contact the local authority social services department, regulator or the police.

> 'If you do make a critical comment in the care home, you can end up being treated as an "interfering relative". Families mustn't be afraid to speak up because they think it could have repercussions on the care of their loved ones. If they don't, nothing will change.' (Family member)

## CONCLUSION: CARE HOMES ARE PLACES TO LIVE!

We do not wish to end this chapter on such a negative note. Care homes, along with dementia care practices overall, have come a long way over recent years. There are many good care homes providing comfortable, pleasant and stimulating places for people with dementia to live. Family members and friends can be assured that their loved ones are being looked after well, and can help enhance the person's well-being by staying involved and supporting the care home's staff.

# CHAPTER 10

# When Dementia Has Become Advanced

## THE CHARACTERISTICS OF ADVANCED DEMENTIA

The final phase of dementia is known as 'advanced' or 'severe' dementia. At this point the person's cognitive difficulties have become profound and are commonly accompanied by increasing physical frailty. Some people can live with advanced dementia in a fairly stable condition for some time, whilst others may progress more quickly. However, as dementia is a life-limiting condition, advanced dementia will eventually lead to the person's death.

The goals of care in advanced dementia are the same as in the earlier years of the condition – that the person has as good a quality of life as possible and experiences well-being. In achieving those goals, however, those caring for the person will need to focus on physical care and supporting the person with activities of daily living to a greater extent than previously. Family members or friends may be undertaking that caring role, or they may be supporting the person in a care home setting. Either way, they will need to come to terms with further changes in their relationship, as the progression of dementia can cause the person to lose the ability to communicate or even to recognise their loved ones. The family will also need to prepare for the person's eventual death. This can be made much easier if the person has made an advance statement, and conversations have been held about end of life before the person reaches this stage. We will discuss this further in Chapter 11.

Advanced dementia usually involves the following symptoms, although families may notice fluctuations, with some days being better than others:

- The person's ability to communicate verbally is increasingly affected. As well as having difficulties expressing themselves, they may appear not to understand language (known as *receptive aphasia*). Their verbal communications may consist of repeated words, phrases or utterances that are difficult to understand. Alternatively, they may be completely non-verbal and just communicate with noises, facial expressions or movements.

- Disorientation becomes increasingly marked. The person may have great difficulty in recognising where they are. They may have limited concept of time. Most significantly, they may also lose the ability to recognise other people, including close friends and family members and even their partner or children. When shown themselves in a mirror or photograph, it is possible they will not recognise themselves.

- Memory loss and cognitive decline also become profound and the person is likely to be able only to carry out very simple activities. Their field of attention becomes reduced and they may be less aware of what is happening around them. Their behaviour becomes limited and often repetitive. A consequence of this is that any previous distressed or restless behaviour tends to lessen, although should still be noted carefully as a possible indication of pain, discomfort or delirium.

- The person is likely to need complete help with activities of daily living, including washing, dressing and eating.

- Control of bladder and bowel function is often affected, and the person can become incontinent of urine and faeces.

- The person is likely to become increasingly physically frail and may lose the ability to walk unaided or be limited to being in a chair for short periods or bedbound.

Faced with such decline, family members and friends may feel estranged from the person, especially if they are living in a care home. Those directly caring for the person may struggle to meet the physical demands and feel uncertain of what difference their support has made. These are pertinent issues, but in this chapter we try to show that people with advanced dementia can have a good quality of life and experience well-being, and families and friends can help them do so.

'My husband had become very acquiescent. He could just about walk about, he had lost much of his speech and he wasn't aggressive towards me. I thought, "I can cope for six months."' (Family member)

'It all depends on what ways I am left with but I would want people to still see me and not my dementia as a priority.' (Person with dementia)

## WELL-BEING AND ILL-BEING IN ADVANCED DEMENTIA

In helping to appreciate what it might feel like to live with advanced dementia, we encourage readers to try the following exercise:

1. Sit back comfortably in your chair and shut your eyes.

2. Take some deep breaths. Focus on your breathing, feeling your breath slowly going in and out, and concentrate on the movements of your chest, rising and falling.

3. After a few moments, slowly open your eyes.

4. Try to imagine you have just woken up and are lying in bed, with no memory of anything that happened just before.

5. Look at your surroundings and any people in the room, wondering how you got there, why you are there and who these people are.

6. Try to imagine what your thoughts and feelings would be if you found yourself in this situation.

What were your reactions to this exercise? Some people may experience emotions such as anxiety, fear or frustration, and thoughts may include 'What has happened to me?', 'Where am I?' or 'What should I do now?' To feel anxious, fearful or frustrated in this situation, you need to have some sense of things having changed for the worse – awareness that there are things that you have forgotten. As we have seen in Chapter 5, people in the early phase of dementia sometimes experience these feelings due to their awareness that their memory is becoming unreliable. In this chapter, however, we are considering advanced dementia, when the person's memory difficulties may have become so profound that they may not remember *anything* – with awareness being only focused on the current moment.

Try to put yourself in the situation described above, and carry out the exercise again.

This time, consider what would influence the way you felt if you woke up remembering *absolutely nothing*.

Some people may feel in this case that their thoughts would not necessarily be negative ones. Feelings may depend on physical factors – such as feeling cold or hot, or comfortable or stiff. Waking up to a quiet, pleasant environment or to lots of noise and glaring light will make a difference. Waking up naturally or how you are woken up is also important. Imagine, for example, being woken by someone roughly pulling your bedclothes off, manhandling you, making loud, harsh, incomprehensible noises and pulling you out of your nice, warm, comfortable bed!

In short, a person's reactions in this situation will depend on how they experience their surroundings through their basic senses. Their feelings will be either positive or negative depending on their level of comfort: how pleasant or otherwise their environment is and how other people interact with them. If all these factors are positive, the person will experience well-being, and if they are negative, the person will experience ill-being. This is the world of someone with advanced dementia. It is a world where the person interacts with their surroundings at the sensory-motor level – experiencing the world through the fundamental senses of sight, hearing, smell, taste and touch and responding with basic 'motor activity'. But the person still has the capacity to have good or bad feelings, and their feelings are going to depend on those around them. If those caring for the person can create an environment that is warm, comfortable and secure, free from stressors and with meaningful human contact, well-being will result.

## RELATIONSHIPS WITH A PERSON WITH ADVANCED DEMENTIA

How can we communicate meaningfully with someone who apparently does not understand language and has difficulty responding to what is being said to them? How can we have any kind of relationship with a person who does not seem to know who we are, even if we are their closest family or life-long partner? When the person reaches the phase of advanced dementia, the contrast between their present state and the way they once were is at its most extreme, and the tendency for family members and friends to feel that 'it isn't really him/her' and to shy away from the person is understandably at its greatest. We may even feel that the person we knew has been 'lost'.

Maintaining a relationship with a person with advanced dementia requires faith that one is doing the right thing and that at some level the person knows that you are there. For many, this is not a problem. The person with dementia is their spouse, partner, mother or father, and they will be there for the person come what may. For others this may not be so easy. But for all who give their time to someone with advanced dementia, the question 'Am I making a difference?' is a pertinent one.

> 'Dad loved mum just as much as he'd always loved her, I know that. When she was in the late stages I can remember him saying, "You'll always be my flower." He'd stroke her and say "It was for better or for worse" and things like that. He never said it was too much.' (Family member)

One way of answering this is to recognise that small successes have enhanced significance. Sometimes with the right environment and care, abilities and functions thought to be lost can return, albeit temporarily. At these times we see a window into the characteristics and person as they once were.

> 'When I brought my husband home and we went through the door, my husband saw the picture on the wall that he'd painted. He gave me a big smile and said "Home"; he hadn't said an intelligible word for months.' (Family member)

## COMMUNICATION IN ADVANCED DEMENTIA

Communication at this stage of dementia is just as important for the person, if not more so, due to their reduced ability to interact with the world. When verbal communication is difficult for a person with advanced dementia, the way we interact without language becomes more important. This includes *para-verbal* and *non-verbal* communication. These are technical-sounding terms for simple concepts.

## Para-verbal communication

This refers to the strategies we use to add feeling or emotion to what we say. It includes such things as our tone of voice, the speed and volume of our speech, the facial expressions that accompany our speech and the other actions or gestures we use. All these things both reflect our emotions and convey our emotions to others – sometimes whether we want them to or not! Through para-verbal means we may convey feelings of happiness, sadness, anger, love, fear, boredom, reassurance and so on.

The relevance of this for interacting with a person with advanced dementia is that the ability to recognise para-verbal aspects of communication often appears to be present after the ability to understand language has been lost. Consequently, a person's sense of well-being or ill-being will be influenced by how we communicate. Recall the exercise earlier in this chapter, when we asked you to imagine waking up with no memory. Compare how you would feel if the first person you came across had an angry expression, and spoke to you in a harsh, loud, unfriendly tone, with your feelings if they had a friendly smile and spoke softly but clearly, with a warm and reassuring manner. Your sense of well-being is clearly more likely to be enhanced in the latter case than the former.

This implies that we continue to talk to the person. Verbal communication is such an integral part of human relationships, and we should never assume that someone with dementia can't understand what is being said. It is possible that they can, even when their ability to respond has been lost. Also, a completely silent relationship (unless one is deaf) does not seem right, and a person with dementia would expect a person interacting with them to speak to them. Finally, the person will often perceive and respond to the feelings that we convey para-verbally whilst speaking to them; without speech, those feelings cannot be properly expressed.

'I don't think my wife recognises anyone now, although I do think she sometimes recognises my voice, but I am not sure she registers who I am.' (Family member)

## Non-verbal communication

The other way we can communicate with a person with advanced dementia is non-verbally. People with advanced dementia may have very limited fields of attention and only be able to attend visually to people or things that are close to and in front of them. Family members and friends will need to be aware of this and use aspects of non-verbal communication to maximise the person being able to attend to them. Sitting straight and looking directly at the person and sitting close to the person and in front of them will help them focus, attend and – perhaps – recognise who is there.

Touch is also a good way of maintaining a relationship with a person with advanced dementia. Often the person seems to respond more to touch than to visual cues or voices. How touch is used will depend on the nature of the previous relationship and what those involved have been used to, but often simply holding the person's hand is an effective way of communicating that you are there for them.

> 'Even though my husband couldn't talk back, we could talk to him. Nothing got in the way to alarm him; he could put all his energies into just living, and I think he was content.' (Family member)

## ACTIVITY AND ADVANCED DEMENTIA

It is tempting to take the view that for people with advanced dementia, activity is impossible, or at least unnecessary. We may feel that the person's communication difficulties, memory loss and restricted field of attention will lead to them being unable to participate in activities in any meaningful sense of the word. By the time that dementia has become advanced, many of the social and diversional activities discussed in Chapter 7 may be beyond the abilities or comprehension of the person. This does not mean that people with advanced dementia have no need of activity or there are no activities that are possible for them. Many people with advanced dementia show signs of wanting to be active, and appear to appreciate it when others help them with activities.

Because cognitive and language difficulties are often so profound in advanced dementia, the best activities are those with less emphasis on intellectual processes and more on the person's primary senses and the involvement of basic actions – what we like to call *sensory-motor activities*. Here are some examples to illustrate the range of possibilities:

- Carol was unsteady on her feet but could walk about with someone to support her. She had lost the use of language and apparently had little awareness of her surroundings. However, when a feather duster was put in her hand, she became much more animated. She went about the room poking her feather duster into corners and across surfaces to clean them, and continued with this activity as long as staff were able to help her.

- Dimitra had also lost the use of language and could not stand unaided. One day a music session was taking place. A nurse offered her a triangle, but Dimitra did not understand what it was for. The nurse then held the triangle up by its string and gave Dimitra the sounding rod. After a while Dimitra got the hang of making a noise by hitting the triangle with the rod, which she proceeded to do continuously. She evidently enjoyed this activity as her face went into the biggest smile the nurses had ever seen from her.

- Henry had always enjoyed sports but was now chair-bound. Nurses tried to engage him in games of 'catch' with a soft ball, but he did not understand the concept of the game. He did, however, enjoy hitting back a balloon that was floated towards him; this simpler activity was understandable to him and engaged his interest.

- Angela was also chair-bound and often appeared tense, sometimes crying out unintelligibly. A staff member who had an interest in complementary medicine carried out a simple hand massage with Angela, using lavender oil. Angela appeared to attend to this activity and for a while afterwards she seemed a bit more relaxed and less inclined to call out.

• Winston had been a dog-lover all his life but was now unable to speak or walk. His family bought him a life-sized soft-toy dog that lay on his lap, and Winston enjoyed stroking and playing with it.

• Eve often waved her hands about and tried to reach out for things. She liked a fibre-optic electric lamp that had a spray of illuminated fibres that waved about and changed colour. She enjoyed stroking the fibres, making them move about, and looking at the resulting light effects.

We could offer many more examples, but these stories help illustrate some basic points about activity with people with advanced dementia:

• Activity is possible with most people with advanced dementia. Most people will retain some awareness of their surroundings, however limited, and want to remain engaged.

• The examples of activity described are linked by their simplicity. All avoid the need for complex cognitive processing and involve basic sensory stimulation or motor actions.

• The gains from such activities are small ones, and the person may only be able to concentrate on them for a short period of time; however, whilst taking part in the activity, the person appears to show enjoyment. Family members and friends should value such small gains – even brief and simple activities are better than no activity.

## NAMASTE CARE

A relatively recent approach being used to support people with advanced dementia is called 'namaste care'. 'Namaste' is a Hindu greeting which means 'to honour the spirit within'. This approach originated in the USA and is now being adopted in the UK in some care homes and hospices but can also be carried out in a person's home. Essentially it involves providing specific interventions that involve the senses. These include activities such as gentle massage, foot spas, music, singing, pets, dolls, nature and offering food and drink. These should be provided in a calming environment, on a regular basis (preferably twice a day), and be shaped according to individual preferences. Some studies suggest this approach can help reduce agitation, distress and withdrawal. Whilst it might be difficult to sustain this in someone's home without extra support, the principles of offering regular stimulation to help maintain communication, engagement and activity are important.

## HELPING PEOPLE WITH ADVANCED DEMENTIA WITH ACTIVITIES OF DAILY LIVING

By the time that dementia has become advanced, the person is likely to be totally dependent on others for activities of daily living such as personal care (washing, dressing and meeting continence needs) and eating and drinking. If the person is living in a care home setting, this help will be provided by care staff, but as discussed in Chapter 9, family members and friends may still sometimes offer assistance, especially at mealtimes. If the person is living at home or in supported housing, care staff may come to the house to carry out particular activities such as getting the person bathed and dressed. In some circumstances, however, family carers may need to develop skills for helping the person with activities of daily living.

## Personal care

Washing and dressing a person with advanced dementia are intimate tasks, and family carers may well feel uncomfortable with undertaking them. The person may not be able to offer any assistance and so the activity must be supported by others. The person may have lost awareness of their need to go to the toilet, or if they are aware, are unable to meet their continence needs themselves or communicate those needs to others.

Giving personal care, including continence care, as well as being embarrassing, can be time-consuming and tiring. Sometimes the person will resist care that is in their best interests. Broadly speaking, there are two reasons for this, both of which can be appreciated by recalling our exercise at the beginning of the chapter. First, as the person's memory and cognitive processes are considerably impaired, they may have little or no conception of what is being done to them, or why. They are aware, however, that others are doing things to their body that they do not understand, but may well find them uncomfortable and feel threatened by them. In those circumstances, resistance is perhaps a natural reaction.

The second reason for resistance is related to the first and stems from the way that those giving personal care go about the activity. Remember in our exercise that we asked you to consider how a person with no memory might feel if they were woken by someone roughly pulling their bedclothes off, manhandling them, making loud, harsh, incomprehensible noises, and pulling them out of their nice, warm, comfortable bed. Some care staff (and perhaps some family carers, especially when feeling stressed) may not appreciate how their manner is likely to be perceived by the person, who will resist if they are approached in the wrong way.

### Principles of giving personal care

If those giving personal care follow some basic principles, this will minimise ill-being in the person, help reduce resistance, and make the experience of personal care a more pleasant one for both the person and themselves:

- Make sure you are well prepared – get everything you need in advance, and keep everything to hand. The person may become more disorientated and distressed if you have to keep breaking off the activity to find things.

- Avoid unnecessary exposure (leaving people uncovered), as this will make them feel vulnerable and unsafe, if not cold! You can help someone wash/dress in stages, leaving only the part of the body you are attending to exposed, or have a towel immediately at hand to cover and keep people warm.

- Use good communication principles throughout. Make sure the person knows you are there before beginning the activity. Talk to them about what you are going to do in a calm and pleasant voice – they may understand what you are saying or at least may be reassured by your tone of voice. Show the person the things you are using (clothes, toiletries, etc.) – they may recognise them.

- Consider using background music as a pleasant distraction to the task in hand.

- Sometimes the person can help a little – encourage them to do so if possible. This can be helped by acting out what you want them to do.

- If the person continues to resist, it can sometimes be helpful to leave them for a while and return later. Always try to keep your temper – as we have seen, the person may well perceive negative emotions and may respond with still greater resistance.

- If resistance is persistent, or the person responds aggressively despite the approaches above, consider if the task really needs to be done or if it can be carried out less intrusively. Would a wash be sufficient rather than a bath or shower? Are there different clothes that are easier to manage?

- Consider if the person is in pain, as this may well explain their resistance. You may need to seek advice from a health care professional about assessment and pain relief. In the meantime, a mild painkiller could be tried, and do things slowly and gently in order to minimise discomfort.

- If the activity has to be done, plan how to carry it out in as safe and dignified a way as possible. Restraining or 'holding' someone in order to deliver care should be seen as a last resort and is covered by mental capacity legislation. Families and care home staff need to be aware of the implications of this, and be careful that any restraint is only carried out 'if it is in the best interests of the person, for the shortest time possible, using the least restrictive approach and only to address the immediate need'. We would recommend no one carries this out alone in order to prevent injury to the person or others, and again, some advice should be sought from a health or social care professional if you feel the person or yourself is at risk.

## Nutrition and advanced dementia

We discussed nutrition, eating and drinking at some length in Chapter 8, and the principles examined in that chapter apply in the same way in advanced dementia. In this phase, however, the person's progressive cognitive and physical difficulties can lead to extra challenges for those caring for them. First, the person may lose the ability to feed themselves, even after trying strategies such as finger foods, and will need others to help them eat. As discussed, in care homes or hospitals, responsibility for ensuring adequate nutrition lies with the nursing and care staff, but family members and friends may want to assist at mealtimes. Sometimes helping a person with advanced dementia to eat and drink is easy, as the person appears to relish their food and readily opens their mouth and swallows. In other cases, more skill and patience is required. Tips for helping a person with dementia to eat and drink include the following:

- Ensure the person is awake and alert.

- Ensure the person is as upright as possible.

- Orientate the person as far as possible, by telling them what you are doing or showing them the plate and cutlery.

- Try helping the person hold the spoon and gently guide their hand towards their mouth.

- If the person doesn't open their mouth, don't assume they don't want to eat. Find a way of assisting the person to recognise that you are offering them food. Sometimes gently putting a spoon to their lips with a little food on it will encourage them to open their mouth.

- Take your time. Don't rush the person or try to give them too big pieces of food, even if they seem to want them. You may risk the person choking or aspiration (see below).

- Make mealtimes pleasant. People with advanced dementia like eating and drinking as much as the rest of us, and a pleasant relaxed mealtime will enhance their well-being. Again, gentle background music can enhance the experience of eating. Use the opportunity for interaction, or at least being with the person in a companionable way.

## Swallowing problems

This is a risk area when helping a person with advanced dementia eat. Many people with advanced dementia may start showing signs of swallowing problems due to the progressive nature of the condition. Early signs can include frequent coughing and spluttering, especially when drinking and/or chewing for long periods without swallowing food. Issues such as poor-fitting dentures, mouth ulcers or tooth pain may be the cause and should be investigated. However, if the swallowing problems persist, a speech and language therapist should be asked to make an assessment.

*Dysphagia* is the term used to describe difficulty with swallowing. A possible consequence of dysphagia is *aspiration*, which occurs when food goes from the mouth into the person's windpipe rather than their oesophagus. In severe cases the windpipe can become blocked, leading to choking, and persistent episodes of aspiration can lead to chest infections, including aspiration pneumonia, which is sometimes a cause of death amongst people with advanced dementia. Dysphagia can result from a number of causes, including the person over-filling the mouth, swallowing without chewing, prolonged chewing or holding food in the mouth. Occasionally the person's swallowing reflex becomes impaired.

The person should be watched carefully when eating for signs of dysphagia and aspiration, which should be suspected if the person persistently coughs or makes a gurgling noise after swallowing. Risks can be minimised if time is taken with meals and the person does not take in large mouthfuls. In some cases, thickening fluids and a soft, fork-mashable or smooth diet may be needed, but pureed food should not be given simply as an easy option.

Another option sometimes considered is for the person to receive artificial feeding, sometimes known as tube feeding, with food being passed down a tube directly into the person's stomach. This should only be considered if there is a realistic expectation it will be reversed, as there are considerable risks associated for people with advanced dementia. Sometimes the tube is threaded down to the stomach via the nose (nasogastric tube (NGT) feeding), or more commonly in dementia care, the tube is surgically passed through the person's skin into the stomach (percutaneous endoscopic gastronomy, or PEG, feeding).

Health care professionals refer to this as 'clinically assisted nutrition and hydration'. If someone doesn't have the capacity to consent to this as a treatment, the same principles of doing things in the best interests of the person should be applied. Those who have a lasting power of attorney for health and welfare must be involved in this decision (see Chapter 5). If there is no lasting power of attorney, family members who know the person well should be involved. In some cases the person may have made an advanced decision to refuse treatment (ADRT) before they lost capacity, and if there is a specific reference to not wanting artificial feeding in this circumstance, this will need to be adhered to. The British Medical Association offers a useful guide for families (see the Resources section at the end of the book).

This is a controversial and emotive issue, as severe dysphagia is often a sign that the person is nearing the end of their life, and studies indicate that PEG feeding can increase the risk of death for people with dementia. As a result, it is rarely recommended. We may also question whether the attempt to prolong life through artificial feeding is justified. We will consider this further in the next chapter.

## When the person becomes incontinent

In advanced dementia, the person may become *doubly incontinent*, meaning that they have lost all control over their bladder and bowel functions, although good practice in helping the person meet their continence needs in the earlier stages may delay the onset of incontinence (see Chapter 8). Once a person has lost control over their bladder and/or bowels, an assessment about the use of incontinence pads should be carried out. Whilst the person is still mobile, the use of elasticated pull-up pads may be the best option to help promote their dignity and encourage independence. Later, when the person is immobile, it is essential that incontinence pads are absorbent enough and fit well. No one should be left for long periods in incontinence pads, and if they become soiled, they should be changed as soon as possible, both discreetly and sensitively.

Whilst it may be tempting to consider the use of a catheter for people who become incontinent of urine, this is not recommended for people in the advanced stage of dementia unless there is an urgent medical need, such as acute urine retention. Catheters can be a source of significant discomfort and distress, and there is an increased risk of urinary tract infections if they are left in place for any length of time.

## Managing pain and discomfort

As discussed in Chapter 8, pain can be a significant cause of distress. Research has shown that pain in dementia often goes unrecognised. Consider that someone in the advanced phase may have limited mobility or movement and may be in one position for a long time. They may have pain from other physical conditions. In addition, they have reduced ability to communicate their pain or discomfort. It is therefore essential that we observe for signs of pain using non-verbal means. There are some specific assessment tools that have been designed for clinicians to help them recognise and treat pain in dementia. Their basic principle is to observe for gestures, facial expressions and noises that might indicate pain or distress especially on movement and when providing personal care. If you notice any of these symptoms, consider pain relief and seek advice.

The main principles of providing comfort in the phase of advanced dementia include:

- Ensuring the person is pain-free through observing their behaviour and giving adequate pain relief

- Maintaining comfort through pressure-relieving mattresses or cushions and gentle repositioning

- Keeping skin clean and dry, through gentle washing, drying and use of moisturising skin creams

- Using well-fitting continence pads and regular changes
- Keeping the mouth moist and clean
- Using aromatherapy, for example, lavender and lemon balm oil or familiar perfumes and air fresheners
- Playing familiar, soothing music or singing favourite songs
- Talking to the person whilst giving care
- Having low lighting
- Having soft textures for the person to hold and touch, such as soft material or toys
- Using touch, including gentle hand massage, stroking someone's face, holding them
- Being with the person and letting them know you are there.

## APPROACHING THE END OF LIFE

The profound cognitive difficulties of advanced dementia, along with increased physical frailty, characterised by progressive issues with mobility, eating and drinking, signify that the person's life is drawing to a close. For some, death may come within weeks or months, whilst others may live on for some years. Sooner or later it will become clear that the person will not live much longer. Those caring for the person will need to make decisions about how the person should be looked after to try to ensure a peaceful death. In the next chapter we will consider care for people with dementia at the end of their life, the role of family members and friends in care and treatment decisions, and also their own needs for understanding and support during this time.

'Having visited the home for two years I have seen other people go downhill and die. I think I have reconciled myself to the fact that my wife is maybe entering that process, that she will die, but who knows how long that will take? Six months, two years, but I don't really want to know.' (Family member)

# CHAPTER 11

# The End of Life

Death and dying are understandably difficult topics for many of us. Nevertheless, dying is a natural process and an important stage for families to recognise, understand and feel prepared for. As we have discussed, dementia is an incurable, progressive and life-limiting condition. This means that all those who develop dementia will die with the condition – it is estimated that one in three people over the age of 60 will die with dementia. Despite this sobering statistic, we would uphold the view shared by Atul Gawande in his book *Being Mortal*, that 'our ultimate goal after all is not a good death but a good life to the very end'.

> 'I want to be able to die with dignity and respect. We need to use the hospice setting far more than we do from point of diagnosis through to end of life.' (Person with dementia)

However, not everyone will die *of* dementia, and not all will reach the phase of advanced dementia before they die. Dementia as a cause of death is often underestimated, though, and as a consequence, the opportunity to provide good end of life care may be missed. In this chapter we consider end of life care for people with dementia whenever and wherever it occurs – people with dementia may die in a care home, in their own home, or in hospital. The end of life may be a time of decision-making, and we discuss the role of family members and friends in those decisions, given that the person with dementia may not be able to contribute themselves. We also consider how family members and friends can support the person in achieving a peaceful death, and how they can meet their own needs for information, support and comfort at this time.

## WHAT IS MEANT BY 'END OF LIFE'?

'End of life' is generally understood as the stage in which people should anticipate the person will die within the next 12 months, including people whose death is imminent (within a few hours or days). Usual indications that someone is reaching end of life include general physical decline, reduced mobility, progressive weight loss, and increasing dependence and need for support. In addition, factors such as repeated unplanned hospital admissions, multiple illnesses and decreasing response to treatments are indicators that end of life may be near. However, as discussed in Chapter 10, some of the symptoms of advanced dementia are similar to the above, and people often show a more gradual decline before they reach the dying phase. This can be difficult for the family as they understandably want to recognise and prepare themselves for the person dying. It is during this time that the most significant decisions need to be reached and supportive end of life care provided for both the person and their family.

The dying phase is the generally quite short period when it is clear that the person's physical condition has deteriorated to the point where death is imminent and is likely to occur within a few weeks or days. Changes indicating the person is reaching this point include:

- Reduced need for food and drink
- Withdrawing from the world
- Changes in breathing
- Becoming increasingly unresponsive
- Changes in skin colour and temperature.

Recognising the dying phase is not an exact science, though, and some of the above may be symptoms of treatable conditions, or of dementia itself. However, if the person has been in the end of life stage for a while and the above symptoms persist, these may be signs that things are progressing.

For some people, being present when the person is dying may be too difficult, and it may be enough to know that the person is comfortable and receiving good end of life care. Others may want to be actively involved. We discuss later in this chapter how families can support people, both during the end of life and at the dying phase.

In cases of sudden death, for example from a heart attack, stroke or accident, there is often no time for the person to experience supportive end of life care. In such cases our attention must be with family members and friends, for whom coming to terms with the person's death can be compromised.

## WHAT CAUSES DEATH AMONGST PEOPLE WITH DEMENTIA?

Death can occur at any time during the progression of dementia. This is due to the fact that the majority of people with dementia are older, with dementia being most prevalent in the oldest age groups. Some people will have developed long-term age-related conditions such as cardio-vascular or respiratory diseases or cancer prior to developing dementia (as we have seen, a history of cardio-vascular disease increases the risk of dementia), or they may acquire such conditions after the onset of dementia. These people may die *with* dementia rather than dying *of* dementia.

With advances in treatment for other conditions, an increasing number of people are reaching the advanced stages of dementia. For these people, death is likely to be as a direct result of dementia as it increasingly affects the functions of the brain.

As mentioned in Chapter 10, people with advanced dementia are often immobile or bedbound, and are at increased risk of swallowing difficulties in which aspiration can lead to pneumonia. In addition, their immune systems are often compromised, leaving them more at risk from chest, urinary or other infections, and less responsive to antibiotics. Vascular conditions such as blood clotting may also be exacerbated by immobility. Sometimes the person simply seems to 'fade away' as the progression of the dementia affects the essential functions of the brain, such as breathing, heart rate and ability to eat or drink.

> 'He recovered from a number of chest infections, with or without antibiotics. On numerous occasions, when the GP came to visit, he would say that he might have a few days, even hours left, and I would call all the family around. It was a roller-coaster of emotions every time.' (Family member)

## FEELINGS OF FAMILY MEMBERS AND FRIENDS AS END OF LIFE APPROACHES

Perhaps inevitably, family members and friends have mixed feelings as they become aware that the person is nearing the end of their life. Sadness and grief at the impending loss is often tempered by a measure of relief that the person's journey through dementia is coming to a conclusion. As discussed earlier, some will have already been experiencing feelings of anticipatory grief, due to loss of the person's abilities and the relationship they previously had. Some will have more or less come to terms with the person's death when the time comes, and may regard it as a 'release', both for the person with dementia and for themselves.

> 'There can be an initial sense of relief and release because the person has become very disabled and you are relieved they are at peace.' (Family member)

Many others, however, will remain devoted to the person and will feel the pain of the impending loss and bereavement regardless of how long the person has had dementia or how far it has progressed. Such feelings may be particularly acute if the person has young-onset dementia and is dying at a relatively early age, but grief is not age-related. Family members and friends must be sensitive to each other's feelings. Saying to a grieving spouse that 'it's for the best' will be of no comfort if the couple has been devoted to each other and the person left behind is devastated at their loss.

## HOW WOULD WE WANT TO DIE?

This may seem to some to be a rather blunt and intrusive question. Death is an uncomfortable subject to many from Western cultures, and speaking about death (or even thinking about it) is still often regarded as taboo. However, reflecting on how we ourselves would like to die will help us understand the issues faced by a person with dementia as they near the end of life, and how to assist them to have the death that they would want. Broadly speaking, we would imagine most people would want their death to include these principles:

- To be told the truth about what is happening to us, so we can prepare ourselves and say goodbye to family and friends.

- To be aware of our medical status and the intended plan of care, such as attempts to resuscitate us if our heart or breathing stopped.

- To die in a place of our choosing. For many of us, this would be our home, but some who are living alone or do not want their families to have to care for them might prefer to die in a hospice, care home or hospital setting.

- To be as physically comfortable and free of pain as possible. If we were unable to do our own personal care, we would want this done in a way that maintained our comfort and dignity.

- To have the option of not prolonging our life if it was clear that the end was imminent, including being able to refuse any treatments we did not wish to receive.

- To be able to carry out religious or spiritual activities if relevant (or have them done for us) and our body to be treated according to our religious beliefs after our death.

- To not die alone. Ideally we would want to be with loved ones when we die, but if that was not possible, we would want to have people with us who had our best interests at heart and could offer comfort and support.

- To know that we were still being watched over and treated with dignity and compassion, if we became unconscious or unaware as death approached.

- For our loved ones to be supported, looked after and comforted, both in the time leading up to our death and following it.

For those who receive palliative care from hospices or palliative care services at the end of life, the above principles may be met, but unfortunately this is not everyone's experience. For people with dementia this will often be even more of a challenge. In the next section we discuss how dementia may compromise the person's experience at the end of life, and how people with dementia may be helped to have as good an experience at this time as is possible.

## DEMENTIA AND END OF LIFE CARE

The opportunity to experience a death that meets the principles set out above can be compromised for someone with dementia as a result of difficulties with communication, awareness and decision-making. Family members and friends often have an important role in supporting the person, ensuring they receive the best possible care and advocating on their behalf. Increasingly, palliative care services including hospices are recognising the importance of offering support to people with dementia at the end of life, and should be considered as an important source of support. Here we consider some of the ways in which end of life care can be supported, despite these challenges.

## Communication difficulties

In advanced dementia, the person's language and communication difficulties will affect their ability to tell others how they are feeling or what their wishes are. It can be particularly hard to tell if the person is experiencing pain or discomfort. Family members and friends may help by using their own knowledge of the person to try to judge their level of pain. Signs of possible pain are increased confusion, agitation or restlessness, changes in sleep pattern, or if the person appears more tense and rigid than usual or vocalises to a greater extent. It is particularly important to observe for signs of distress when the person is being moved which might indicate pain, such as grimacing, moaning, tears or protective body postures. Such changes should be reported to medical or nursing staff, who should respond by using medication to relieve pain or other means of enhancing comfort.

As discussed in Chapter 10, it is important that the person is communicated with. It is likely that the person may comprehend at some level, and will feel reassured by family members' and friends' presence.

## Awareness

Are people with advanced dementia aware at this time that their life is coming to an end? In most cases it is impossible to answer this. Symptoms of advanced dementia will often have resulted in less awareness of surroundings, and as we have seen, indicators of the dying phase additionally include withdrawal and becoming increasingly sleepy or unresponsive. It may, indeed, give us a degree of comfort to think the person is not aware they are dying.

We must, however, always assume that the person may have some awareness of their surroundings and that they need comfort and support. The person's religious or spiritual preferences should be respected and gone through, even if the person is not apparently aware of any ritual or ceremony taking place. Family members and friends may need to advocate on behalf of the person with professional staff – or each other – if they feel that the person is not being treated with due respect or proper care is not being given.

## Decision-making

If the person lacks mental capacity at end of life and doesn't have an advance care plan, their wishes about care and treatment at the end of life may not be known or acted on. In Chapter 5 we discussed the importance of making advance care plans whilst the person is still able to indicate their wishes. This may include an advance decision to refuse specific treatment (ADRT) at the end of life, an advance statement and/or wishes expressed within a health and welfare lasting power of attorney (LPA). However, if this has not taken place, the family still has a crucial role in ensuring decisions are based on the best interests and wishes of the person.

Research shows that the majority of people want to end their lives in familiar surroundings, and most do not want to die in hospital, although a large number of people in the UK do end their lives in hospital. For people with dementia this may be due to family carers feeling unable to continue to care for the person at home at the end of life, an acute health crisis that can't be catered for, or sometimes due to a lack of resources to provide proper nursing or medical support in the person's home. Increasingly, care homes are caring for people until the end of life, although this depends on staff having the skills and resources to care for dying people and advance care plans being in place. With the right support and a shared understanding of the person's wishes, emergency admissions to hospital, which may result in an undignified death, can be avoided. Whilst hospital admission may be in the person's best interests in some cases, advocacy by family members and friends may allow the person to end their life in a more appropriate environment, cared for by people who know and respect them.

Treatment or care decisions that may need to be taken include whether to attempt to resuscitate the person if their heart or breathing stops; whether to use artificial feeding in cases of swallowing difficulties; or whether to give drugs or other treatments that might prolong the person's life. As mentioned, if the person has drawn up an ADRT related to these areas, that decision would be legally binding, so long as it was properly drawn up and unambiguous. Alternatively, the person may have appointed a family member or friend as their attorney, to make care decisions on their behalf. Without such formal arrangements having been made, family members and friends have no legal power to make decisions for the person, but good practice holds that doctors or nurses should consult family members when such decisions have to be made. Ideally this will have taken place before the last stages of life are reached.

'During my husband's last chest infection, he looked weary; he couldn't hold up his head any more and his swallowing went completely. He was on a very low dose of oral antibiotics, and the doctor asked if I wanted to have him brought into hospital to have intravenous antibiotics and hydration, or if I wanted to keep him at home and let nature take its course.' (Family member)

## Do not attempt resuscitation (DNAR) decisions

In the UK, if the person is in hospital and a DNAR decision has *not* been made, staff are obliged to attempt to resuscitate a person whose heart or breathing has stopped. Resuscitation can be undignified and uncomfortable for the person, and is considered much less likely to be successful for people with advanced dementia. Even if the person survives, they may experience further health problems and crisis situations before their eventual death.

DNAR decisions can only be taken by a doctor, and family members or friends cannot direct doctors either to resuscitate the person or otherwise. The person themselves, through the medium of an advance decision, can, however, express that they do not wish to be resuscitated in these circumstances, and doctors should, in most cases, respect that wish. This should also be the case if the person has appointed an attorney for health and welfare and given the attorney authority to make such decisions.

At the same time, DNAR decisions should not be automatically made for all people with dementia who have serious illnesses. Resuscitation can prolong life, and if the person has early dementia, they may experience many more good quality years if they recover from physical illness. We would oppose any health care system that discriminated against people with dementia by denying them treatment simply on the grounds that they had dementia – all such decisions should be taken in the best interests of the person, not the health care system.

## Artificial feeding

As discussed in Chapter 10, artificial feeding is sometimes proposed for people with advanced dementia who, towards the end of life, develop difficulties with swallowing. This is a highly controversial treatment in this context. Whilst current advice does not suggest a blanket ban on artificial nutrition and hydration, neither nasogastric tubes nor PEG feeding are recommended for the end of life. It is argued that there is no evidence that artificial feeding improves the person's strength and abilities or reduces pressure sores at this stage. In addition, introducing a nasogastric or PEG tube is uncomfortable and undignified for the person and leads to less contact with others through eating and drinking. Complications may arise if the tube becomes infected or dislodged, or if the person pulls it out. Although the person may not take in much food orally, lack of desire to eat is common at the end of life, and the person is likely to die of the underlying disease process rather than from starvation.

These seem to be powerful arguments against tube feeding and the procedure is rarely applied nowadays, but family members and friends may be consulted regarding its use. A person drawing up an advanced decision may wish to express their view regarding whether or not they would want artificial feeding if they had advanced dementia, or advise a person acting as their legal attorney accordingly.

'I had to reassure the care team that now my husband could no longer swallow we would not be starving him to death because in the dying process he would feel neither hungry nor thirsty, provided his mouth was kept moist and clean.' (Family member)

## SUPPORTING PEOPLE WHO ARE DYING

There are number of ways in which a person can be kept comfortable during the dying phase, and family or friends may find it helpful to contribute to someone's care and offer comfort. Here we address these in relation to the changes people may experience.

### Reduced need for food and drink

When someone starts to die, their body no longer has the same need for food and drink as before. This is because the body's metabolism slows down and becomes less able to digest food. Although people may stop drinking and their mouth can look dry, this is not necessarily a sign that they need to drink. Ways to help can include:

- Wetting their lips with a damp sponge

- Applying lip balm

- Offering small sips of fluid, if appropriate.

## Withdrawing from the world

In advanced dementia, people often spend more time asleep, and their withdrawal may be gradual. In the dying phase this may become more apparent, with less and less time spent awake and the person becoming less responsive. If the person is comfortable and pain-free, this can be a calm and tranquil time. Ways to help can include:

- Spending time with them

- Touching their arm or holding their hand

- Speaking to them, even if they don't respond, so they can hear the tone and sound of your voice

- Playing gentle music, especially any that the person previously liked.


## Changes in breathing

Breathing can change at the end of life and can become more shallow, irregular or noisy due to the mucus that settles in people's throats. This can feel distressing to watch but it is, in fact, just a sign that the body is slowing down. Ways to help can include:

- Changing the person's position to help move the mucus, if breathing is noisy

- Medication suggested by palliative care specialists or doctors. This is usually given through a syringe driver (via a small needle inserted into the arm) and is called *anticipatory medication*. It can help with reducing the build-up of mucus, but also includes medication to reduce nausea and anxiety and provide pain relief.


## Becoming increasingly sleepy/unresponsive

As the person's body starts to shut down, the person is likely to become less responsive, and you may notice changes in the person's colour or skin as blood circulation reduces. This is usually quite peaceful but occasionally someone may become more alert or agitated. This will usually be short-lived, but if prolonged, you should ask for advice about medication to ease the distress. Ways to help include:

- Staying with the person and trying to offer reassurance through talking or holding their hand

- Remembering that this is a normal process, and just being there will offer the person comfort.

## A GOOD DEATH?

Consider the following true story, as related by Michael, a care assistant in a nursing home:

> James had been resident in the home for about six months but he had become very disabled and completely dependent. He'd been a stockbroker by profession. His wife visited him a lot but he didn't seem to recognise her; he just mumbled to himself when she was there. Then he weakened markedly and it seemed clear that he would not live much longer. He was unable to eat solid food, and was fed through a feeding cup, though with difficulty. One afternoon at teatime, I brought James his drink and prepared to help him. He looked at me intently and seemed to be trying to communicate with me. He said in a low, distinct voice, 'No...no...' I took the drink away. That evening James died, peacefully, with his wife by his bedside.

What do we make of Michael's story? Do we believe that James was actually trying to communicate his real wish, and what do we think of Michael's decision to go along with that apparent wish and take the drink away?

Some writers have related anecdotal evidence of what have been termed *intermittent spontaneous remissions*, brief occasions, usually near to the end of life, when people with advanced dementia have had apparently lucid moments and have seemingly been able to communicate with others in a meaningful way. Was this one such moment? And if it was (or if it wasn't), did Michael do the right thing by not giving James the drink?

It is highly unlikely that Michael hastened James's death by his decision, and we may perhaps regard what he did as a humane individual act. Good care for people with dementia at the end of life is essentially the same as good care at every phase of the condition. The principles we have promoted throughout this book, of person-centredness, flexibility and treating people with dementia as individuals worthy of respect, apply as much at the end of life as at any other time in the person's journey through dementia.

> 'At the end we took positions of holding and cradling him and he just stopped with the rattling, strained noise and it eased off to normal breathing. The breaths got further and further apart, and he just slipped away – it was very peaceful.' (Family member)

## SUPPORT AFTER DEATH

The ability to provide comfort and well-being at the end of someone's life can be of particular concern as it is a memory many people are left with after the person has died. For those who are unable to achieve this due to circumstances out of their control, there can be an overriding sense of guilt and loss. In contrast, if we are able to ensure that the person has received the best care possible, this can be replaced by feelings of satisfaction and reassurance.

After the person with dementia has died, family and friends continue to need support. The loss of a close relative or friend with dementia can have the same impact in terms of loss and bereavement as anyone else, even if it is anticipated and comes as a relief that the person is no longer 'suffering'. As with any death or loss, practical arrangements for the funeral can keep people occupied initially, and often during this time others are on hand to offer support and help. However, once this is over, there can be a gap left, especially for those who have been very involved in providing care, whether at home or through regular visits to care homes. Some people have referred to delayed bereavement. Family and friends should try to continue to support each other, and bereavement counselling for those who are significantly affected may be a useful form of support.

'Sixteen months after my husband died this bereavement shock hit me like a sledgehammer, and I didn't know what was happening to me, both physically and mentally; I still haven't really got it sorted yet.' (Family member)

# Conclusion – Suffering from Dementia or Living with Dementia?

'So-and-so is suffering from dementia.' How often have we heard or read that phrase? We don't need to spell out its implications. The person is 'suffering'; they are experiencing anguish, ill-being and poor or non-existent quality of life, and by extension, their friends and family are too. Such phrases are part of the negative stereotype of dementia that the media still portrays.

We have included quotes from a number of people who are 'living with dementia' or, as Wendy Mitchell (an author herself) comments, 'living as well as possible'. These people have actively embraced their diagnosis early on in the condition and have found valuable sources of support and activity to help maintain their well-being. They are all also active campaigners who wish to change the negative view about dementia that sometimes pervades the media, to ensure that people with dementia have rights in the same way that other people with disabilities are entitled. As we know, though, attitudes can take a long time to change.

We occasionally read about well-known people or celebrities who have dementia and most likely they too will be described as 'suffering' from the condition, but by no means are all people with dementia 'suffering'. Take, for example, the American pop singer and guitarist Glen Campbell. Early in 2011, at the age of 75, he was diagnosed with Alzheimer's disease, having experienced memory difficulties for some years. Instead of slipping out of the public eye to 'suffer' with his condition, he embarked on a world concert tour, singing his famous songs to audiences of thousands and playing guitar as well as he did in his youth. Look him up on YouTube and you will find excerpts from some of those concerts. What stands out from those clips is that far from 'suffering', he is having a whale of a time. He's making the best of the time he has left, and is a classic example of someone *living with dementia*.

Another example is that of George Melly, the British jazz musician and singer who died in 2007 at the age of 80. George was diagnosed with vascular dementia yet continued to do live concerts until a few months before he died. With his wife Diana he made a film about vascular dementia and its impact on people with dementia and carers.

Of course, neither Glen Campbell nor George Melly could achieve these things unaided. The help and support received from family and friends was vital. In the case of Glen Campbell, three of his children played in his band, to support and guide him on stage, and his family was proactive in promoting his well-being. He used autocues to help him remember the song lyrics. George Melly was ably supported by his wife and by long-standing band members who were able to provide cues for familiar songs. With such assistance, their quality of life and sense of well-being were maximised – and they could continue to give fans pleasure as well.

We trust that our readers will recognise in the stories above some of the themes and ideals of this book, and that they will engender in readers the hope that their own journey through dementia, for all its trials and difficulties, will not all be suffering. Family members and friends, with professional assistance, can make a big difference to the lives of people with dementia, and when the journey is over, they can have the satisfaction that they have helped the person to *live* as well as possible with dementia.

# Resources

This section provides contact details for non-profit and government organisations that provide information about caring for people with dementia and offer support to family members and friends. Information given here is taken from the organisations' websites.

Age UK, the UK's leading charity working with and for older people, includes information and advice about money, care, health or housing for older people:

Advice line: 0800 678 1602

www.ageuk.org.uk

Alzheimer's Disease International, worldwide federation of Alzheimer's associations, supports people with dementia and their families:

www.alz.co.uk

Alzheimer's Research UK, the UK's leading dementia research charity, includes information about dementia and research developments:

www.alzheimersresearchuk.org

Alzheimer Scotland, the leading dementia organisation in Scotland, campaigns for the rights of people with dementia and their families and provides an extensive range of innovative and personalised support services:

24-hour Dementia Helpline: 0808 808 3000

www.alzscot.org

Alzheimer's Society, a UK care and research charity for people with dementia and their carers, provides information and support, improves care and funds research:

National Dementia Helpline: 0300 222 1122

www.alzheimers.org.uk

Dementia UK, a charity that provides Admiral Nurses, specialist support for families affected by dementia, includes information, advice and resources about dementia and caring:

Admiral Nurse Dementia Helpline: 0800 888 6678; email: helpline@dementiauk.org

www.dementiauk.org

The Lewy Body Society, a charity that funds research and raises awareness of Lewy body dementia, includes information about the disease and advice for those affected:

www.lewybody.org

NHS Choices, About dementia, information provided by the NHS about dementia, including causes, symptoms, diagnosis and treatment, with links to other useful resources:

www.nhs.uk/conditions/dementia/about

Young Dementia UK, a dedicated national charity for younger people with dementia and their families, includes information and resources:

www.youngdementiauk.org

## CHAPTER 1: BECOMING FAMILIAR WITH DEMENTIA
### Dementia in seldom-heard groups

Culture Dementia UK is a charity that supports carers and people with dementia from the African Caribbean community:

www.culturedementiauk.org/about

Dementia Alliance for Culture and Ethnicity (DACE) is an alliance of groups currently providing information and support to people from Black, Asian and minority ethnic communities in the UK:

www.demace.com

National Dementia Action Alliance (NDAA), From seldom heard to seen and heard, information about a campaign focused on those with dementia and learning disabilities, dementia within prison settings and dementia within the LGBT+ community:

https://nationaldementiaaction.org.uk/campaigns/from-seldom-heard-to-seen-heard

Young Dementia UK provides information and support for those affected by young-onset dementia:

www.youngdementiauk.org

## CHAPTER 2: BEING A FAMILY MEMBER OR FRIEND OF A PERSON WITH DEMENTIA
### Children and dementia

Dementia UK provides a range of information, videos and resources for children, young adults, parents and teachers about dementia:

www.dementiauk.org/get-support/children-young-people-and-adults

## CHAPTER 3: SOMEONE CLOSE TO ME MAY HAVE DEMENTIA
### Diagnosis and treatment options for dementia

Alzheimer's Society, Diagnosis:

www.alzheimers.org.uk/about-dementia/symptoms-and-diagnosis/diagnosis

Alzheimer's Society, Treatments:

www.alzheimers.org.uk/about-dementia/treatments

Dementia UK, Getting a diagnosis:

www.dementiauk.org/understanding-dementia/getting-a-diagnosis

NHS Choices, How to get a dementia diagnosis:

www.nhs.uk/conditions/dementia/diagnosis

NHS Choices, What are the treatments for dementia?:

www.nhs.uk/conditions/dementia/treatment

### Rarer forms of dementia

Alzheimer's Society, Rarer types of dementia:

www.alzheimers.org.uk/about-dementia/types-dementia/rarer-types-dementia/

Rare dementias, information and support provided by University College London, Dementia Research Centre about rarer dementias, including familial Alzheimer's disease (FAD), fronto-temporal dementia (FTD), familial fronto-temporal dementia (fFTD), posterior cortical atrophy (PCA) and primary progressive aphasia (PPA):

www.raredementiasupport.org

## CHAPTER 4: SOURCES OF SUPPORT FOR PEOPLE WITH DEMENTIA AND THEIR FAMILIES AND FRIENDS

Admiral Nurse Dementia Helpline: 0800 888 6678

www.dementiauk.org/get-support/dementia-helpline-alzheimers-helpline

Alzheimer's Society, Dementia Talking Point, an online community for people with dementia, carers and families:

https://forum.alzheimers.org.uk

Alzheimer's Society National Dementia Helpline: 0300 222 1122

www.alzheimers.org.uk/get-support/national-dementia-helpline.

DEEP, The UK Network of Dementia Voices, engages and empowers people living with dementia to influence attitudes, services and policies that affect their lives:

www.dementiavoices.org.uk

Dementia UK, How an Admiral Nurse can help:

www.dementiauk.org/get-support/admiral-nursing

tide: together in dementia everyday, the UK-wide network for carers, and former carers, of people living with dementia:

www.tide.uk.net

## CHAPTER 5: THE EARLY YEARS OF DEMENTIA

Dementia UK, Advance care planning documents:

www.dementiauk.org/understanding-dementia/advice-and-information/planning-ahead/planning-now-for-your-future-advance-care-planning

Dementia UK, Life story work:

> www.dementiauk.org/for-professionals/free-resources/life-story-work

## Assistive technology

Alzheimer's Society, Using technology to help with everyday life:

> www.alzheimers.org.uk/get-support/staying-independent/using-technology-everyday-life

AT Dementia provides user-friendly information on assistive technology for people with dementia, including what is available and how it can be obtained and used:

> www.atdementia.org.uk

## CHAPTER 6: MANAGING CHANGE AS DEMENTIA PROGRESSES

Mental Health Foundation, What is truth? An inquiry about truth and lying in dementia care:

> www.mentalhealth.org.uk/publications/what-truth-inquiry-about-truth-and-lying-dementia-care

## Disability aids for people with dementia

Alzheimer's Society online shop, Daily living aids:

> https://shop.alzheimers.org.uk/daily-living-aids

Disabled Living Foundation, Living Made Easy, comparison site for independent living equipment:

> www.livingmadeeasy.org.uk

Unforgettable, a website 'to improve the lives of all those affected by dementia and memory loss':

www.unforgettable.org

## CHAPTER 7: SOCIAL AND LEISURE ACTIVITIES AS DEMENTIA PROGRESSES
### Ideas for keeping active
Alzheimer's Society, Activity ideas for people with dementia:

www.alzheimers.org.uk/get-support/staying-independent/activity-ideas-dementia

Social Care Institute for Excellence, Keeping people with dementia active and occupied:

www.scie.org.uk/dementia/living-with-dementia/keeping-active

## CHAPTER 8: THE CHALLENGES OF DEMENTIA
### Aromatherapy
Dementia UK, Aromatherapy:

www.dementiauk.org/understanding-dementia/advice-and-information/complementary-therapies/aromatherapy

### Music
Age UK, Dementia and music:

www.ageuk.org.uk/information-advice/health-wellbeing/conditions-illnesses/dementia/dementia-and-music

Dementia UK, Music therapy:

www.dementiauk.org/music-therapy

Playlist for Life:

www.playlistforlife.org.uk

## Reminiscence

Social Care Institute for Excellence, Reminiscence for people with dementia:

www.scie.org.uk/dementia/living-with-dementia/keeping-active/reminiscence.asp

Unforgettable blog, What is reminiscence therapy?:

www.unforgettable.org/blog/what-is-reminiscence-therapy

## General hospital care

Alzheimer's Society/Royal College of Nursing, This is me, a simple leaflet for anyone receiving professional care who is living with dementia or experiencing delirium or other communication difficulties:

www.alzheimers.org.uk/get-support/publications-factsheets/this-is-me

National Dementia Action Alliance (NDAA), Dementia-friendly hospitals:

https://nationaldementiaaction.org.uk/campaigns/dementia-friendly-hospitals

## CHAPTER 9: CONSIDERING RESIDENTIAL CARE FOR PEOPLE WITH DEMENTIA

### Funding residential care

Age UK, Paying for residential care:

www.ageuk.org.uk/information-advice/care/paying-for-care/paying-for-a-care-home

Alzheimer's Society, Care home fees:

www.alzheimers.org.uk/get-support/legal-financial/care-home-fees

Paying for Care, Helping you plan how to pay care fees:

www.payingforcare.org

## Guide to care homes

Carehome.co.uk, a guide to over 18,000 care homes, nursing homes and residential homes providing care in the UK, and also the leading UK review site for care homes:

www.carehome.co.uk

## CHAPTER 10: WHEN DEMENTIA HAS BECOME ADVANCED

### Resources for managing health

Dementia UK, information leaflet on maintaining health in dementia:

www.dementiauk.org/understanding-dementia/advice-and-information/maintaining-health-in-dementia

## Artificial feeding and dementia

British Medical Association, Clinically-assisted nutrition and hydration (CANH):

www.bma.org.uk/advice/employment/ethics/mental-capacity/clinically-assisted-nutrition-and-hydration

## CHAPTER 11: THE END OF LIFE
### Recognising dying

Dementia UK, Understanding dying, understanding the changes that happen when someone is reaching the last days of their life:

www.dementiauk.org/understanding-dementia/advice-and-information/planning-ahead/understanding-dying

# Index